SLEEP

EXACT BLUEPRINT on How to Sleep Better and Feel Amazing

Brain Health, Memory Improvement & Increase Energy

Table of Contents

Introduction

Life today seems to move faster than it ever has. Every hour is consumed with so many tasks, it's almost as though we never really rest. Even when we lay down in our beds at night, the pace of the world around us intrudes, when we should be resting up for the next round with our fast-paced lives.

If you're reading this, I'm sure you know the drill. Your head hits the pillow and you think, "I'm tired. I can't wait to sleep". And just as that thought crosses your mind, others follow it.

"Did I lock the front door? Did I pay the electricity? What about that doctor's appointment I have to take my mom to? Are the kids really sleeping? I'm not looking forward to that meeting tomorrow!"

Even though we know we're ready to sleep, we can't seem to will ourselves into a state of relaxation that allows us to fall into the kind of sleep we need. Tense and anxious about the demands of our lives, we lay awake at night, counting worries instead of sheep; checking off items on our "to do" lists, instead of becoming one with our pillows.

Then there are the realities of living in the 21st Century that go beyond the pace of our modern lives. The incessant light, for example. Have you ever gone into the wilderness and slept in a tent? Have you ever spent the night in a rural inn, or farmhouse?

If you've had one of these experiences, or something similar, you'll remember how remarkable the darkness was. Almost palpable, it enveloped you as you lay in your sleeping bag, or bed. If you live pretty well anywhere in the world, though, artificial light is a constant reality. Streetlights and the ambient light you find illuminating the night in any place humans live, are ubiquitous.

Then, there's the noise. The world is ever in motion, as cars and trucks whizz down the roads and highways. Even if they're off in the distance, you can still hear them. In major cities, add car alarms and the hum of transformers and other white noise. It's never quiet. It's never dark. You can't turn it off and you can't turn your mind off, either.

How on earth is one to get a decent night's sleep?

The human animal needs, for optimal functioning, Rapid Eye Movement (REM) sleep. This is the kind of sleep typified (as the name suggests) by rapid movement of the eyes under the lids, colorful and vivid dreams and extreme relaxation in the muscles of the body. REM sleep normally accounts for approximately 20% of the total sleep cycle. While we all get it, even if we're suffering from sleep disturbances, it's possible we aren't getting nearly as much as we need due to this problem.

That's what this book is intended to help you with. I want to provide you with a blueprint to move toward sleeping more soundly and, in doing so, feeling amazing! You may think a good night's sleep is something you'll never know, but there are so many techniques and strategies to ensure a peaceful night's sleep, you'll probably be surprised.

Let's explore the world of sleep together, talk about some common challenges and then walk through effective solutions to the problem.

Before we can get to understand how to improve your sleep, it is very important that we ask ourselves this important question; how do you stand to benefit when you get enough sleep? In simple terms; what's in it for you when you get enough sleep? Let's learn more on this in the first chapter.

Chapter 1: The Benefits Of Getting A Full Night's Sleep

With all of this talk about how to sleep better, you might be wondering what exactly makes sleep so special. After all, it is essentially remaining unconscious for a few hours right? You may think that sleeping less would allow you to do a great many things with your life as you would finally have time on your side. However, sleep has a number of benefits. This chapter is dedicated to informing you about the various benefits that getting a full night of restful sleep can provide.

1. **It Boosts Happiness**

Now that safety and food are no longer a major concern for most people, we have started to focus on more abstract desires and needs, such as the need to be happy.

Many people are unhappy these days. We work more than we do anything else; everything is a race and the way the world is run induces a constant sense of hunger so that we consume as much as possible. It is fair to say that the average person right now is quite miserable.

However, there is a major reason that people are unhappy that has nothing to do with any of those things: we are not getting enough sleep.

Sleep is where we deal with the emotional issues that we cannot deal with in our waking state. Dreaming allows us to rationalize our fears and desires; it allows us to get over our frustrations.

Sleeping also helps your body repair itself. If your body doesn't get enough rest, it will end up getting damaged and causing you pain. A lack of sleep also makes it difficult for your brain to regulate itself, thereby resulting in an imbalance that can affect your mood.

In fact, research has shown that lack of sleep affects mood even more than low income.

2. It Makes Sex More Fun

Sleep is one of the most important processes that your body goes through. While sleeping, one of the most important activities that the body is able to conduct is the regulation of hormone levels within the bloodstream.

One of the hormones that it regulates is testosterone and its female counterpart estrogen. These hormones are primarily responsible for sex drive. If your body is healthy and is maintaining the secretion of these hormones, you should have a normal sex drive and should enjoy sex.

Not getting enough sleep, on the other hand, means that you are going to have fluctuating levels of testosterone or estrogen in your body. The most immediately noticeable result of this is a sudden drop in sex drive.

Not getting enough sleep also results in a number of other sexual dysfunctions as well. Erectile dysfunction is quite common among people who don't get enough sleep, for example.

By getting enough sleep, on the other hand, your body will be completely healthy and ready to have sex, and since your body is chemically balanced the sex is going to feel a lot better too.

3. It Helps you Get Buff

It may seem odd, but by sleeping right you are actually going to make it a lot easier to get muscular. This has a lot to do with what your body does while your brain is asleep.

While you are asleep, one of the most important processes that is going on within your body is the repairing of your muscles. Over the course of the day, your muscles invariably get damaged in one way or another. If nothing else, they get worn out from being used for so long. While you are sleeping, your body is able to repair the damage and get your muscles ready for the next day.

This becomes especially important if you are working out and trying to build muscle. The soreness you feel after an intense workout is actually caused by microscopic tears that develop in your muscles when they are overworked.

Your body responds to this by rebuilding the muscles and then overcompensating, making the muscles larger and stronger so that they can take the strain of your workout. It does all of this reparation and regeneration while you're asleep.

However, if you do not get enough sleep, you are going to notice that your body simply won't be able to build any muscle. No matter how much you workout, your muscles won't be getting that much bigger. You will also notice that it is taking your body far too long to get over that post workout soreness.

In fact, not sleeping enough for an extended period of time can potentially result in muscle atrophy. This means that your muscles will actually start to shrink in size because your body is not getting enough time to repair them.

Hence, if you want to build some major muscle, keep in mind that the best way to do that is to get enough sleep every night.

4. It Makes Your Mind Sharper

You have probably noticed that pulling all nighters is not a very good idea. In fact, a lack of sleep in general makes you a lot less mentally sharp, often making even the simplest of tasks feel impossible if they require you to use your brain.

This is because when your mind is deprived of sleep, it loses a significant portion of its cognitive abilities. Your brain needs a particular balance of chemicals in order to perform at maximum capacity. Neurons firing are a lot like electricity. If the wiring is faulty, the electricity won't pass through properly.

This is exactly what happens to your brain if you do not sleep enough. Your brain repairs and rejuvenates itself while you sleep, preparing it for mental challenges that it might have to face one day.

If you are experiencing difficulty performing tasks that require you to think, try sleeping more. You will be surprised at how much your mental performance will end up improving after you have been getting a full night's sleep for a few nights in a row.

5. **It Prevents Car Accidents**

It is a commonly accepted fact that driving home drunk is extremely irresponsible behavior. This is because your judgment is impaired, along with the fact that you are drowsy and thus can get confused and drift off of your lane. There are several reasons why driving drunk is unacceptable.

All of these reasons apply to driving while sleepy as well. Driving while sleepy is particularly dangerous because if you are very sleep deprived you can end up suffering from instances of micro sleep. Micro sleep would be a moment of unconsciousness that does not last more than two or three seconds. If this happens while you are driving it can result in catastrophic accidents.

Sleep deprivation can result in a number of other phenomenon as well, such as double vision and delayed reactions that can potentially result in deadly crashes as well.

If you are well rested, your judgment is going to be greatly improved, and there will be absolutely no chance that you would veer off of your lane. Staying well rested is an important part of being a responsible driver, just as important as not driving while you are drunk.

6. **It Helps you Lose Weight**

This is another fact that may seem odd to you. After all, while you're sleeping you're basically just lying there, doing nothing whatsoever. By this logic, getting up early and working out for longer could help you lose more weight.

However, this logic is ignoring one extremely important point: sleep is necessary in order to keep metabolism up. Metabolism is the process by which your body utilizes energy. Having a high metabolism is one of best ways to lose weight. Some people are born with high metabolisms, but these become useless if a regular sleep schedule is not maintained.

If you don't get enough sleep, your body will slowly become unable to maintain processes like the metabolisms of fat. This is why it is highly common for people who do not get enough sleep to be obese.

In fact, a lack of sleep is one of the most common causes of obesity. No matter how much you work out, it will all be useless if you are not giving your body and mind adequate time to shut down and regulate the various functions they are responsible for. If you can't seem to lose weight, chances are it's because you're not getting enough sleep.

7. **It Reduces the Risk of Diabetes**

For a lot of people, diabetes is in their genes and thus will certainly develop at some point in their lives. For other people, diabetes can develop due to environmental factors. Whatever the case may be, getting enough sleep is one of the biggest ways in which diabetes can be prevented.

Even if the disease is in your genes, if you are getting enough sleep you are going to be able to postpone the disease indefinitely as long as you monitor your diet and take regular exercise as well.

Sleep helps with this because of the role that it plays in the regulation of hormones in the body. The lack of the hormone insulin is what causes diabetes. If you are getting enough sleep, your body will be able to keep the pancreas health, thus ensuring that you get more than enough insulin.

However, if you are not getting enough sleep every gland in your body is going to suffer, including the pancreas. If your body is not getting enough rest, it will start to malfunction. Once your pancreas starts malfunction, you will have started suffering from diabetes and there will be no way to reverse it.

8. It Helps Relieve Stress

You might have noticed that you always feel better after a good night's sleep, no matter how terrible the stress you are trying to overcome is. There is a very important reason for this.

Apart from regulating hormone levels and allowing the body to repair itself, sleep allows your brain to overcome things that are making you anxious. You might have bad dreams while you are asleep, but when you wake up you will definitely be feeling better.

If you are stressed out, chances are that your brain needs relief even more than usual. Sleep allows your brain to turn itself off and essentially prepare yourself for stress. This is why people who have been emotionally charged and stressed for a long period of time tend to crash and fall asleep rather quickly. Sleep allows the brain to repair itself and protect the mind from permanent damage.

Stress often prevents sleep, but if you have a pre-sleep routine that is strong enough, there will be nothing that can stop you from sleeping. Once you wake up, you will find that whatever was bothering you seems a lot more manageable.

9. It Helps you Make Better Decisions

Sleep deprivation leads to two distinct changes in the chemical composition of your body. Firstly, the level of serotonin in your body decreases. Additionally, your body starts to secrete more adrenaline, believing that you staying up is an important part of your survival and secreting chemicals to help you do it.

This has a huge impact on your decision making skills. Serotonin has a leveling influence on you. It allows you to gauge a situation for what it really is in a calm and collected manner.

Adrenaline, on the other hand, forces you to act quickly. It is traditionally released during a fight or flight response, and is thus designed to help you make decisions without thinking too much about them. This can be useful in situations where your life is in peril, but otherwise it is not a very good trait to possess, particularly when you are making decisions that require thought and consideration.

The loss of the leveling influence and the presence of something, which makes you impulsive means that not getting enough sleep will have you making rash decisions. Get enough sleep so that you are able to make good decisions after careful consideration.

10. It Will Help You Save on Medical Bills

Chances are, a large chunk of the chronic illnesses you are suffering are caused by sleep related disorders. The lack of sleep can wreak some major havoc on your body, and if this extends over a long period of time the problems can become serious and even result in death.

In order to keep ourselves healthy, we usually end up spending a great deal of money. Doctors are expensive, particularly if you are suffering from a serious illness. Hence, medical bills are a regular worry for a great number of people, and often play a major role while making a budget for the rest of the month.

You will be surprised at just how much you will be able to shave off of your medical bill by getting enough sleep. Heart problems, diabetes, muscle atrophy even balding can be prevented if you get an adequate amount of sleep throughout the night.

If your doctor bills are making it difficult to save any money, try upping the amount of sleep you get each night by an hour or two. You will be able to see results within days!

11. It Makes You Less Likely to Abuse Substances

Alcoholism and drug addiction are two major problems that affect a lot of people. However, there is an underlying cause for these addictions that might surprise you.

Although this is certainly not true for everybody, a lot of people become naturally inclined towards substances abuse if they are not getting enough sleep. This is because a lack of sleep ends up disrupting your circadian rhythm. One of the major results of this disruption is a twisting of the reward system of the brain.

Since you are lacking in sleep, your brain will feel less pleasure than it would otherwise. Most people are perfectly content with their lives even if they are facing hardship. If you lack sleep, on the other hand, you are going to find it difficult to remain content.

In order to compensate for this, you might end up drinking too much, or possibly even start taking drugs. There is no excuse for alcoholism and drug abuse, but if you are finding yourself drawn to these activities, try to ascertain whether you are getting enough sleep or not. A month of getting regular, quality sleep might remove your desire to lean towards such destructive activities entirely.

12. **It Helps Prevent Headaches**

A lot of people suffer from various kinds of headaches. One of the most common types of headache is the migraine. There are a variety of other common headaches as well, such as cluster headaches. Whatever the type of headache is, lack of sleep exacerbates it.

If you suffer from regular headaches, changing up your sleep pattern might help a lot. Your brain would achieve a more stable chemical balance that would facilitate a lower incidence rate for headaches. This is particularly effective for migraine headaches. A lack of sleep can often result in severe migraine headaches that can get so painful that they end up being debilitating, preventing the person suffering from them from moving.

Another one of the most common causes for headaches is stress. Stress causes the muscles in your neck to tense up, which ends up putting strain on your cranium and causing major headaches. By sleeping more and sleeping better, you are going to allow your body to relieve itself of unnecessary stress. As a result, your headaches will subside in a domino effect, which is in turn going to help you, sleep better as well.

13. **It Boosts Your Immune System**

This is perhaps one of the most significant benefits that a regular sleep schedule can provide. The problem with not getting enough sleep is that your body gets fewer resources to conduct renovations. One of the places where your body takes resources from in order to compensate for this shortfall is your immune system.

You won't suddenly become susceptible to major diseases and die, but chances are that if you don't get enough sleep you are going to end up getting diseases like the common cold and the flu more often.

A lack of sleep can also make you more susceptible to infections. Even cuts that aren't so deep could end up getting infected and causing you to fall ill. This can be particularly dangerous if you have been deprived of adequate sleep for a long period of time. Your immune system would be particularly weak in this situation, making it very possible that an infection could get out of control.

If you find yourself falling ill frequently, getting more sleep could reduce the instances of illness. People who get enough sleep rarely ever fall ill, and if they ever do they hardly stay ill for very long.

14. **It Will Make You More Patient**

This is another important benefit of getting enough sleep. Lack of sleep causes severe irritability. This is actually a defense mechanism put in place by your brain. Since it is not functioning at maximum capacity, it starts looking at certain things as threats even though they are not really threatening in any way. This is why you start reacting aggressively for no reason when you are sleep deprived.

Serotonin, a chemical your body is deprived of while you are sleep deprived, plays a major role in making you patient. Adrenaline kicks your survival response into overdrive, and is produced in excess while you are sleep deprived. Hence, you become extremely irritable if you haven't gotten enough sleep.

If you start getting enough sleep, you will notice that your patience will increase. Fewer things will annoy you, and when you do get annoyed you will be able to ignore it instead of overreacting or making a scene.

Sleep may seem like a waste of time if you look at it as simply being unconscious, but with benefits like these, it's clear that it deserves to be a priority. With all the benefits that come with getting enough sleep, you would expect that many of us would be getting enough sleep or at least trying to. Unfortunately, that's not what has happens for many of us.

Chapter 2: A Common Problem

You're not alone. The Centers for Disease Control and Prevention report that an estimated 50 to 70 million Americans suffer from lack of sleep. Worldwide, almost one quarter of the worlds working people experience difficulty sleeping.

Stress at work, family worries, financial woes and relationship problems are high on the list of reasons so many of us struggle to get the sleep we need. The CDC typifies difficulty sleeping as a public health problem, due to the impact of sleeplessness on society as a whole. Sleeplessness can be responsible for accidents (including those on the road and in the operating theatre) and serious occupational errors. Nodding off at inappropriate times (at work, at school, while driving) and trouble concentrating are common problems seen in those who aren't sleeping well at night.

It's also worrisome that a lack of sleep can lead to health problems in those suffering from it. Diabetes, obesity, hypertension and even cancer can be provoked by a lack of sleep.

Most people need between 7 and 9 hours of sleep each night, but since 1942, the amount of sleep most people in the United States get is only 6.8 (an hour less than the 1942 average). This point to a diminished quality of life for those who aren't getting adequate sleep.

But why? What is it that's keeping us up at night?

Stress

Researchers at the Harvard Business School and Sanford's Graduate School of Business recently published a report that found that workplace stress is responsible for as many as 120,000 deaths per year, in the USA alone. In addition, researchers identified a cost of up to $190 billion in health care expenses attending this dire statistic.

Our lives have not only become busier, but much more sedentary. This is particularly true of office jobs. Add to this the constant worry in our lives about everything from job stability to family integrity to bills waiting to be paid, and you have a recipe for health disaster.

However, stress is not always unhealthy. A little stress presses us forward, helping us get done what we need to get done and to achieve our goals. A completely stress-free life would bear little fruit. There's a line, though, and when that line is crossed, your sleep and health can be severely impacted.

When stress prevents us from resting adequately, there is a cascading effect in our lives. Irritability, depression, sluggishness and inattention can all lead to life consequences in our families, relationships and workplaces.

What's The Stress Point?

Your first move towards addressing stressors in your life that are preventing you from getting the rejuvenating rest you need, is to identify what's really eating away at you.

Researchers at KJT Group, Phillips, discovered that the most common stressors related to sleep problems were money and work. 28% of respondents in the study cited economic concerns as the factor that burdened them with the greatest amount of stress. 25% said work was their most stressful life reality.

This won't be news to many of us, but perhaps asking ourselves if these are the thoughts that keep us awake at night is a start. Sometimes, life's ups and downs are carried into our beds at night, preventing us from getting the rest we need.

Are you overtaxed at work? Do you have a physical pain issue? Is there a looming problem in your life you need to take positive steps toward addressing?

So What Should You Do About It?

- **Don't hold it in.** Talk to someone close to you. Taking the time to tell a friend or family member that something's bothering you can help to lighten your load. Take the time to write down the pros and cons of situations that may be bothering you. Be orderly in your financial affairs. Be diligent in living within your means, to the best of your ability. If your job is keeping you up at night, maybe it's not the right job for you. Taking stock of situations weighing on your mind is the first step toward addressing them effectively.

- **Make time for self-care.** Use your breaks at work to disengage from what you're doing. Go for a walk. Sit quietly somewhere and look out through the window. Go and get a cup of tea. If you can avoid it, don't work through your breaks. Take them and use them as your oases in a busy day.

- **Where does it hurt?** Go and ask your doctor if there's a health issue more serious than an ache or pain. Engage yourself in an activity that relieves the pain, like swimming or yoga (more on these below in the "Exercise" section). Don't suffer in silence; it will only add to your stress. Share it with a professional who can help.

- **Be kind to yourself.** You are not a failure because you can't manage everything that gets piled on you. Maybe you're so accommodating that people come to you first when there's something they want done. Maybe it's time to address that. Learning to say "no", when appropriate to your needs and the work you're doing, is not a sign of weakness. It's an act of self-preservation. Embrace "no". Identify allies in your workplace willing and able to help and then, call on them.

- **Trouble on the home front?** Don't stew about it; act. Talk to your errant child, your irritable spouse, or whomever it is the problem is emanating from. Tell them how you feel. Not addressing the problem is causing it to grow in your mind, when it may be nothing at all, or something you can fix with a heart-to-heart, or the drawing of a boundary. Communication is your friend and leaves a better taste in your mouth than "stew".

- **Work smart, not hard:** One principle of effective time management is to do high quality work as opposed to high quantity work. The best way to do this is to concentrate on the results and not how busy you are. Just because you spend a lot of time, doing something does not mean that you will achieve better results. Similarly, staying an extra hour at your work may not be the best way to manage your time at the end of the day. Chances are you will feel resentful about working after hours. In addition, there is a high probability that you will be less productive, which will make you even more frustrated and compound your stress.

- **Do a good prep:** You'll have to admit that there's nothing stressful than being unprepared. You need to be organized for tomorrow, spend some time making your to do list and cleaning up before you leave. If you have everything covered up, you're less likely to fret about work when the night or evening comes. After you come in the following morning, you'll be relaxed to be in total control and able to handle things. Being prepared sets a positive tone for your day, and allows you to accomplish more things.

- **Prioritize:** Both men and women do worry but women tend to worry in a more global way. Men do worry on something specific or actual but women worry abstractly concerning their weight, job, or health status of a relative. However, try to keep your stress or worries focused only on real and immediate issues, and fight those that you have zero control on them. Organizing your worries can help you reduce the stress overload.

- **Manage Your Time:** It's not unlikely and unheard of that you may get overwhelmed by the list of things you have to do. This may obviously be a cause of stress. It's a fact that you can't manage everything all at once unless you make schedules that are easy to follow. Begin by making a list of the things you want done based on priority. Also, categorize the list based on what you should do personally and what can be delegated to other people. Note those tasks that should be done immediately, those to be completed by the end of the day, next week or forthcoming week. The key here is to classify or manage big tasks into manageable tasks spread over some time, and delegating those that don't demand your personal attention. When managing your time, create buffer times where you can address emergency or unexpected tasks. Also have some time to relax and restore your well being.

- **Say 'No':** This is important when you have too much to do over a little period. Learn to say "No" to unimportant requests or additional tasks that can overwhelm you and cause stress. The sad thing is that majority of people can't manage to say "No" as they might appear rude and self-centered. However, be aware that barriers to this issue are self-created and can be overcome with a friendlier tone. Adopt a few humble expressions such as:

"I'd love to do this, but …"

"I'm quite busy now. Can you ask me again at….?"

- **Take Control:** Some situations that cause worries, stress, and anxiety don't really mean that they are impossible to solve. Learn to look for remedies to your problems so as to feel in control and reduce stress. If unsure of how to begin, write down the problem and then brainstorm as many possible solutions as you can. Then pick each solution and analyze the good and bad side of it to realize the safest and reliable solution. Highlight each step that you require to undertake to solve the problem, i.e. what to do, how to do it, when to complete and who to be involved.

- **Keep a regular journal:** Synchronizing your body's sleep wake cycle is a very effective strategy to achieve good sleep. Set a fixed bedtime and wake up time to ensure you get the same amount of sleep every day, even on weekends. You can take a nap to make up for lost sleep, instead of waking up late in the morning. This way, you can cover up for lost sleep without interfering with the sleep-wake pattern. How do you know if you are getting enough sleep? If you find yourself awake before the alarm feeling focused and mentally sharp, then you have slept enough.

- **Have a lunch break**: Most busy people tend to work through lunch break in a bid to get more work done. This is generally not a good idea, and can even prove to be counterproductive. It is generally agreed that taking at least thirty minutes off from your work will improve your productivity in the afternoon. Taking a break gives you a chance to relax and take your mind off work. You can take this time to do some exercise or go for a walk. You will get back to your desk feeling rejuvenated with renewed focus and a new set of eyes. You can even plan your day using a midday break to help you break up your work into manageable bits.

- **Try the "4D" method**: Attempting to do all tasks requested through your email might at the end make you feel unproductive, frustrated, and tired. It has been shown that more and more workaholics today are experiencing some form of email stress. The first decision you make when you open an email is very crucial when it comes to addressing work addiction. To effectively manage this burden, you may want to use the "4 Ds" model to make your decision:

-Delete: You can probably delete almost half of the emails you receive immediately

-Do: This applies when the email is urgent or when it can be dealt with quickly

-Delegate: If someone else can deal with the email better

-Defer: Schedule some time to deal with the email if it requires longer action

All these problems are manageable with some reflection on your part. In the whirlwind of our busy lives, we too often pretend there's no time to reflect; for introspection. But this is one of those tales we tell ourselves to perhaps avoid those internal dialogues that need to be conducted.

How Much Sleep Do You Really Need?

Sleep is very important and everyone makes a conscious effort to get enough of it to feel fresh and less tired. However, you could be living a highly productive life or having an insanely busy schedule. With numerous responsibilities, you're forced to economize, slice up your working time and try to balance between tasks. Based on research, 90 percent of people can function better after 7-9 hours of sleep. A further 3 to 5 percent may function normally after less than 6 hours of sleep while only 1 percent of people sampled could manage less than 5 hours of sleep.

Most studies have shown that lack of sleep has a number of side effects. It disrupts normal body systematic functions right from metabolism to the immune system. Insufficient sleep can also trigger health conditions such as mood disorders, memory problems, attention deficit disorder, low fertility, obesity, and heart disease. On top of these physical symptoms, extreme fatigue can make you less alert and more prone to impulse behavior, memory lapses, and inability to fight stressors.

Apart from the medical problems, sleep deprivation makes you less efficient at work, and lowers your ability to solve problems, make decisions, communicate effectively, be innovative, and adapt to situations. Despite this, around 1 percent of the people can manage to work efficiently on about 4 hours sleep without serious side effects. "Short sleepers" are people who have genetic mutations that allow them to thrive in busy environments and work all through.

What matters is the amount of time you sleep within 24 hours as opposed to the sleep you average during the course of a night. If you cannot manage the 7-9 hours of sleep daily, you can choose to take a few 20-minutes naps while in the taxi, at work or other place. Even if the 7-9 hours of sleep are recommended for your physical health, remember to balance with the health of your career. In most times, you have a tough deadline to complete tasks and it's worth it to stay up late till it's done.

My rule of life?

Time is not something you have. It's something you *make*. It's worth your while to carve out at least an hour a day to tackle the little things we too often let slide. Instead of tuning out in front of the television, tune in to some of the life details crying out for your attention.

Busy. Busy. Busy.

Go here. Go there. Do this. Do that. Pick up the kids. Pick up the groceries. Pay the bills. Have a social life?

If you feel there aren't enough hours in a day, you're certainly not the only one. In our over-stimulated, 24/7 culture, it's increasingly difficult for people to slow down long enough to realize just how fast they're going.

Slowing down to take stock of things; to enjoy life, is something few of us make a point of finding time for. We are over-scheduled, overtaxed and worst of all, over tired.

But no matter how tired we are, so many of us have difficulty getting the quality sleep we need and our modern day "busyness" is a big part of the problem.

The hectic pace of our lives can come between our pillows and us. American sleep scientists have discovered that people who experience poor sleep quality often "sleep snack". When their bodies are given an opportunity to slow down, even for a moment, they doze off. Sleep-deprived, this clear message from their bodies is saying, "I need a good night's sleep!"

But brief periods of rest like "sleep snacks" don't solve the problem. They're no substitute for the good night's rest you need to be at your most alert and effective.

If You Can't Beat The "Busy", Manage It

Those of us who work at home are especially vulnerable to work invading other sectors of our lives. Where does work end and the rest of your life begin? For those who work at home, it's a tough call. Even those of us who leave our homes every day to go to work often don't park that part of our lives outside the front door when we walk through it at the end of the day. The emails keep coming. The phone keeps ringing. Loose ends demand tying up. In some ways, 21st Century communication portals have not made our lives easier. They've just made our work lives more able to intrude on time with family and friends.

Drawing boundaries is a balancing act. Telling those you work with you're not available after a certain hour is sometimes seen as a declaration of disinterest. Nobody wants to hear from their boss in the middle of the night, but sometimes it happens. Varied time zones, emergencies and contingencies happen at midnight just as often as they do at 4:30, or 5:00 pm, when you're ready to leave for the day. Beyond such urgencies, you are in charge. Drawing boundaries is a process that should begin as early in your working relationship as possible. Don't permit a situation that encroaches on your personal time to continue for months, or even years on end. Doing so is as good as telling your boss or co-workers it's OK with you.

It's not OK to expect you to be available 24 hours a day. Whenever possible, be clear about your boundaries in this respect. Instead of accommodating every demand, try saying something like:

"Thanks for calling on me. I'll be on this first thing in the morning."

You've quietly drawn a line in the sand. At the same time, you've acknowledged the importance of the request with the kind of language you've employed. In addition, you've shown appreciation for the trust placed in you. Try it. It works.

The demands of others don't mean you're not in control of your time. You are. Slowing down is about more than drawing boundaries for others, though. You have to draw them for yourself, too. Take an honest look at how you spend the "spare" time you have. What do you do to relax?

Is it actually relaxing, or is it just one more thing keeping you plugged in, busy and frayed around the edges?

Does it keep you awake at night, as your mind struggles to shut down and sleep?

Time management is a discipline that can be applied to every area of your life. If done intentionally and with integrity, you'll find there's time in your day for everything you need to do, including spending time with your family and friends. There's even time for you.

Here are some life hacks to get you started:

If You Leave The House To Work:

- **Lay out your work clothes the night before**. Make sure everything you're taking from your closet is clean and ready to wear. This will prevent last minute scrambles to locate a tie with no stains on it, or a snag and run-free pair of pantyhose.

- **Coming home at night, change your clothes.** Put them in the closet if they're still good to wear. If not, put them in the laundry. How many Saturdays have you spent picking dirty clothes off the floor, because that's where you threw them when you came home? Get your partner and/or family in on the act. The time you spend picking up clothes and putting them where they're supposed to be is now yours.

- **Flaking out on the couch** is something most of us like to do sometimes, but laying there night after night, with the television watching over you as you look passively on is not only a waste of your time, it's another source of noise. So many of us turn the television on the minute we walk in the front door each evening. Advertisements, the superficial news cycle, meaningless reality shows – these are not enriching your life. Reduce your viewing time gradually. Choose what you'll watch. If there's nothing on you find appealing, turn the television off. Use the time you'd usually spend passively receiving information you don't need doing something you enjoy. Go for a walk! Visit with a friend! Take up a hobby! Using the time consumed by television to make space for the activities and people you love, will bring you greater peace and better rest.

- **Reduce the time you spend on social media.** As we all know, platforms like Pinterest and Facebook can consume countless hours of the time we need to slow down and get back in touch with what we love about our lives. Have a purpose when you open your social media account. Say what you want to say. Share what you want to share, but don't spend countless hours scrolling when you might be soaking in your tub, taking a much-needed, restorative bath. Start by scheduling and limiting your time. As you begin to wean yourself off these time-consuming activities, you'll find you've replaced them with options that serve you and your wellbeing much more effectively. Like television, there are many empty calories involved. Use the time you've been spending on social media for something that nourishes you, instead!

If You Work At Home:

Telecommuting is an option a growing number of people turn to. Conventional wisdom may lead us to believe that working from home frees more of our time. It's often the case, though, that working in the home is rife with distractions and opportunities to squander time. On the other hand, some who work from home log more hours and find it difficult to detach from their working lives.

Many of the life hacks mentioned above apply to people working at home just as readily, but here are a few specially tailored to those who telecommute:

- **Schedule yourself.** Get up at the same time each day and follow an agenda. You can always re-organize for contingencies, but sticking to an overall "shape" is a good way for stay-at-home workers to remain focused.

- **Make a list** of what you want to accomplish during the course of your day. You might want to do this the night before. That way, your goals are already set and you can hit the ground running.

- **Head off temptation** by being disciplined as to when and for how long you take your breaks. Take these often. The time you'd spend commuting, waiting for the bus, dressing for the office, packing a lunch – all this is time you can use to get away from your laptop and do something to clear your head (how about a little exercise?).

- **Don't procrastinate.** Meet your deadlines and complete your deliverables by resisting the urge to involve yourself in household matters in the time you've allotted for work. There is time for those, but not when you're working. Work when you've scheduled yourself to work. Attend to other matters when you've completed your work for the day.

Honestly assess how effectively and efficiently you manage your time and ask yourself what else you can tweak to clear away time to address details you normally can't seem to get to. There is time in your life. There is ample opportunity for you to "unbusy" yourself.

You just need to sit down, map out a course of action that fits your lifestyle and make the time. When you discover all those hidden hours, you'll be astounded. You'll also feel less taxed, stressed and pushed up against the wall, because you have become the master of your time. You've created the space you need to feel more relaxed about the demands of life.

You have *taken back* your time! Achieving this is crucial to feeling more centered in your life.

Chapter 3: Boost Your Day's Sleep

Although there are 24 hours in a day, most of them are already reserved for other activities that do not include restful sleeping. You often get tempted to work overtime or until after midnight even against your natural sleep patterns. But regardless of how hard it is to rest after each long day, be aware that each night's rest is a non-negotiable priority. You therefore must be efficient and use the 24 hours we have in a day to the best of your ability. This is the only way you can completely rest and refresh your bodily processes.

That said what should you do to ensure that you get a continuous cycle of high-quality sleep. The only guarantee to ensure that you sleep soundly is to maintain a friendly routine soon after you wake up, during the day and soon before you get to bed. Simply by devoting minimal time to the actual preparation of sleeping, while focusing primarily on getting quality sleep every night, you can get the rest you need to live the life you've always wanted with more energy and passion every day.

The following steps can help you perform better and still obtain sufficient sleep under a strict timeline:

When You Wake Up In The Morning

There are few measures that you can take to ensure you get quality sleep the night or day ahead. However, the most recommendable and effective strategy is to try sleeping in different phases. Scientists developed a concept referred to as Polyphasic sleep, where you simply break up your sleep into multiple short blocks as opposed to one long single block. For instance, you can choose to be biphasic sleeper in that you sleep shorter durations daily. You can decide to wake up at 8 AM, get into your schedule until lunch, get into another 2 hours nap, and continue to work until 2 AM. This concept also allows you to take 20-minute naps every 4 hours, though this can become complicated or difficult to follow.

To utilize sleep-in-phases concept, you only need to adapt flexible schedules that can help you get into regular nap routines that suit your working schedule. To develop one, be aware that good quality sleep shouldn't involve use of over the counter medication in order to influence your body's natural functions or senses. You don't have to force sleep or attempt to fall asleep more quickly, but it's a healthier thing to wake up easily, energized and feeling more refreshed.

If you rarely manage a minimum of 6 hours of sleep at night, a more recommendable routine is to take a 20-minute afternoon nap in your office. Try setting a timer for 20 minutes and then briefly lie on the couch with an eyeshade. Since taking medication isn't a good idea, try doing meditation or other mindfulness exercises such as repeating a single mantra as you inhale. For instance, you can choose a mantra like "happiness", "love", "peace" or pick other phrases that best describe you. With these steps, majority of people have managed to fall asleep and wake up naturally after 20 minutes even without a timer.

If you find napping in your office rather strange or unprofessional, you can inform your employees, work counterparts or other people that you'd take a longer period at the coffee outlet. However, this might not work always as per your script. Sometimes you may have to stay up late or probably awaken earlier by your kids. That's why you should follow a regular routine while in the office, or take naps in other random places such as in the car as you wait to pick your kid up. For example, you can take a 15 minutes nap at 8 AM as you drop kids to school, another short nap at 11 AM and later 15 minutes in the mid-afternoon.

The main idea is to get asleep as soon as you feel fatigued or tired as this helps you sleep faster and thus maximize productivity. There are times you'll need to work up the entire nights but you can find ways of extending your schedule. When very busy in the house, take 20-minute naps on your couch for every 2-4 hours, which should total to at least 1 hour of sleep time. With a 3-4 nap schedule, you can manage to work up overnight and still manage to wake up fresh and less tired, albeit for a few days.

- **Be appreciative**

One of the worst things about waking up early is the negative effect it has on your emotions. You wake up feeling groggy and grumpy and do not want to talk to anyone. It is important to take some time when you have just woken up to reflect on your life, otherwise you will go through the rest of the day with that ugly feeling. When you wake up in the morning, take some time to reflect on the things in your life. Give thanks for your work, your family, and friends in your life and realize how different your life would be without them; Be grateful for your wife or husband, for your kids, and for your boyfriend or girlfriend. Do this through meditation i.e. take a few deep breaths, each time bringing into picture the person you are grateful for. Let this person sink in with every breath you take, then say a little prayer for the person; or just bless them. Simply being grateful puts your mind in a positive attitude. This attitude helps you wake up feeling nice and warm and motivates you throughout the day.

- **Reward yourself**

You might find that waking up early in the morning can be terribly dissatisfying because of the early morning drowsiness you experience. You sometimes wake up tired and even feel sleepy; sometimes, you end up giving up and falling back to bed. This is because you have not set the appropriate goals that will super boost you out of bed immediately that alarm clock starts to ring. Setting a reward for yourself when you wake up motivates you to get up and puts you in a better mood than waking up without any motivation. When you are motivated, you are likely to be more productive and enjoy your day than when you are not. It does not have to be a great deal per se, but just something to keep you going.

You can achieve other benefits with this strategy. Another great advantage of rewarding yourself in the morning is that it helps instill discipline needed to wake up early in the morning. When you know that there is a reward in waking up early, you do your best to go to bed as early as possible so that you wake up early. When you have accomplished your goal of waking up early throughout the month, you will be happy because of your achievements, and will even enjoy your reward happily. Here are a few ways you can reward yourself in the morning:

1. You can promise yourself a gift when you wake up at the exact time your alarm rings for the whole week.

2. You can put your coffee maker in your room. That way, you can reward yourself with a cup of coffee when you wake up to start your system.

3. Watching a morning show or news can also be a great source of motivation to get you started.

During The Day

There are also steps that you can undertake during the day to facilitate good sleep that day especially if you have a busy schedule. The worst thing is when the simple steps you want to take fail to make sense! For instance, sometimes after a busy day, you may need to take a few naps to relieve tiredness or tension but soon you become wide awake and frustrated. The bad side is that lack of sleep during this stipulated period may cause involuntary sleep in the course of working time.

Nevertheless, you need to be creative here. Let's say you have a very busy schedule like strict deadlines to observe, tasks to perform and other demanding responsibilities. On the positive side, obtaining a 20-minute restful sleep can help rejuvenate you and calm your anxious mind. However, if you have a hard time sleeping during the mid-morning or afternoon break, you need to learn how to nap.

Different people may feel an urge to take the occasional nap anytime during the day. But the majority of people often feel like napping at around 3-5 PM when their energy levels have dropped. You need to take a couple of naps with each no longer than 20 minutes, as exceeding this time might leave you unsteady or unable to fall asleep later in bed. Knowing your sleep patterns can help you lighten the mood, boost your productivity, and feel better.

To understand your sleep patterns, keep a sleep diary to help you track your thoughts, daily habits and sleep patterns. It's easy to establish the time you go to bed, how long it takes to get a nap, whether you wake up before morning and when you wake up. This is very important for busy people and new moms who have an erratic sleep schedule. Experts advise people to avoid napping after 7 hours from getting up from bed. In case you feel sleepy, try napping early, but not 7 hours after waking up as this can mess your sleep routine. Such disruption can cause you to sleep late and thus wake up late as well.

In The Evening

Regardless of the amount of work or tiredness making you anxious, you have to get ready for a sweet and peaceful sleep. These few techniques can help you get prepared a few hours before getting to bed:

- *Converse with yourself*

The main factor that hinders effective sleep is stress. That's why you need to concentrate your mind to yourself in order to help drain stressors of life. Talk to yourself silently on topics that don't create stress. For instance, talk about what you'd like to carry on tonight. Also try to dialogue with your inner self about your dreams or aspirations.

- *Play a game*

Another way to calm down the mind is to play a few mindful games such as counting your breath. When in your office and unable to play games, take advantage of the rhythm and monotony of counting as this can soothe your mind. You can also count sheep, and focus on maintaining the sheep jumping a fence. The little level of concentration in this game can create enough stimulation to work up late or sleep better.

You can also choose to play real games, such as crossword

puzzles or solitaire. For real games, place the game material where you can easily assess them, and under low light. I would recommend that you try out solitaire since the game is repetitive, not demanding and requires concentration with less mental effort. However, if you want to reduce screen time or avoid the blue light, playing the card version can help you relaxed compared to the computerized version under bright light.

During the Night

Do you want to start your day well in the morning? Then ensure that you get the right amount of sleep the night before. If you do not get enough sleep, you will wake up feeling tired, grumpy, and sleepy. The rest of your day will be less productive and you will be more vulnerable to accidents because of lack of concentration. When you have determined the right amount of sleep you need, create a routine so that you go to bed and wake up at the same time every day.

Train your brain to prepare to sleep by creating a sequence of habits before going to sleep. You can start by taking dinner, having a shower, reading a book, listening to some music and then going to bed. Here are a few steps to help you get enough sleep during the night:

- **Pray**

Different people have distinct beliefs. Regardless of your belief, it's important to say a little prayer before going to sleep. Praying helps to relax your mind by focusing and letting go of your worries. Prayer works in a similar way as meditation. If you do not pray when you go to sleep, are tensed, and worried, the stresses accumulated through the day can haunt you in your sleep. You will sleep uncomfortably because you are worried what tomorrow will be like.

Studies have shown that many cases revolving around insomnia are caused by stress. As such, when you pray, you put your mind to rest and forget the stresses affecting your life. Prayer can help you feel at peace right before you go to sleep. When you are praying, your mind relaxes and helps you let go of your day's worries and stresses, making it easier to sleep. You also enjoy a good night's sleep when you pray because you have faith that you are at peace and that nothing can scare you because you have a super natural being watching over you. This helps you to have a good night's sleep, free from nightmares and restlessness.

Thus, before you tuck yourself to sleep, make sure that you are in a state of peace and calm. If necessary, take out your spiritual book of your choice then read a few verses to help you meditate and relax. After reading the verses, keep calm and close your eyes to pray. Say a short prayer about the things affecting your life. Then you have to believe that all your problems are under control, and then jump to bed. Majority of believers often report experiencing improved sleep after regular practice of prayers.

- **Cool down:**

Do you struggle to sleep and find yourself wriggling uncomfortably in your bed? This could be because of the temperature in your room. Being in a room that is either too hot or too cold makes it hard for your body to achieve the internal temperature set point that your brain is accustomed for you to fall asleep. For instance, high temperatures can affect you in several ways. For instance, you become sweaty or restless, and eventually wake up. Therefore, before going to sleep, achieve the ideal temperature for your room by following these simple guidelines:

1. Set the optimal temperature: The ideal temperature your room needs for a good night's sleep is around 19-21 degrees Celsius. Adjust the thermostat in your air conditioner to meet that range. Getting your room to the temperature range of 19-21 degrees Celsius helps your body reach this temperature faster.

2. Allow Air in the house: On a hot day, close the curtains and blinds to prevent sunlight, and open them when the sun is setting. Open the windows too to let in that cool evening

breeze into your room.

3. Install a fan to help maintain the room cool. The general idea is to make your room cooler so that your body reaches the set point temperature faster. Getting a fan helps to eliminate excess heat that may make it uncomfortable to sleep.

- **Relax**

To get a good night sleep, it's vital for you to be relaxed. Keeping your mind at rest is the key to getting a good night's sleep. Being prepared to sleep helps your mind get rid of any disturbances, especially by taking big breaths and visualizing. When you are in a relaxed state, your mind takes time to slowly take in the day's activities and consolidate any new things learnt without tension. This way, you are able to enjoy a good night's sleep and wake up feeling refreshed in the morning that follows.

On the other hand, when you are not relaxed before going to bed, chances are high that you will not get a good night's sleep. You will be restless at night, twisting and turning before you go to sleep. Your dreams can also be affected if you go to sleep when you are tensed; or worse still experience nightmares in your sleep! Here are a few steps to help you out:

1. Stop doing any work at least one hour before going to bed to help your mind settle before sleeping.

2. Use some breathing techniques outlined here to help you relax. Take a few breaths, hold your abdomen and chest for a while, and then breathe out. Repeat this exercise a few times.

3. Train your brain to sleep with a sleeping routine. Set a specific time to go to bed as well as waking up.

4. Make your room as comfortable as possible. Let your brain know that your room is meant for sleeping and sex only by getting rid of any work related materials on your bed. Let it be dark by turning off all the lights.

5. You can take advantage of your diary, or just a small

notebook to write down the things that happened that day, your achievements and so on. This will help to clear your mind and obtain relaxation.

6. Write down any problem that may be causing tension in your life now. Also write any possible solutions on the same paper and then throw it away with your tension.

7. Visualize: imagine you are in a place of peace and tranquility. Use your senses to feel the place and consequently relax your mind.

Note: While what we've covered so far is very helpful in getting you to sleep, you can still benefit a lot more by learning some more specifics that will get you to sleep without trouble. Let's discuss this in detail in the subsequent chapters.

Chapter 4: Using Your Time For Optimal Sleep

Now that you've mastered time management, I hope you've taken some of the suggestions about how you use it to heart. These suggestions are just the beginning. So are the changes you've made. As you see the fruits of your efforts, you'll start to address other areas that need similar attention and before you know it, your life will be the finely tuned masterpiece you've always dreamed of living.

With the time you've found, you've already taken an important step towards better sleep because you've made positive changes. By taking control of your time, you're already more at ease. Stress and feeling burdened to the breaking point will most certainly have diminished because of the positive steps you've taken.

Can you feel that? It's the peace you've just cleared space in your life for and that peace is the doorway to better sleep.

Now let's talk about the sleep enhancement practices you can pursue with at least some of this extra time.

Exercise

It's a dirty word to some. But did you know it's one of the most important things you can do to improve not only your overall health, but also the quality of your sleep?

Dr. Christopher Kline, of the University of Pittsburgh points out that while many are aware of the impact of exercise on sleep, science is only now making definitive connections between the two. While it's common knowledge that physical activity can tucker you out, the scientific community is still uncovering why that is.

In 2013, the US National Sleep Foundation's study found that those who engaged in vigorous physical exercise reported sleeping soundly twice as often as those who didn't. In addition, Dr. Kline's recent work has revealed that sleep apnea (when breathing stops during sleep) sufferers who are assigned an exercise regime routinely experience an improvement in symptoms. This was also found to be true in subjects suffering from obesity. Even if the exercise assigned didn't result in significant weight loss, its effects on sleep apnea and sleep quality were seen to be considerable.

But the US National Sleep Foundation has also found that the timing of exercise can have an impact on how you sleep. For example, exercising at night can actually lead to decreased sleep quality. Exercise raises your body temperature and your body can take up to six hours to cool down. Optimal sleep depends somewhat on temperature (a factor we'll discuss later on in this book). Being overheated before bedtime will only add to your woes. It's therefore suggested that late afternoon is the best time for exercise.

The Foundation also relates that their studies have revealed that getting 150 minutes of exercise a week (a little more than 20 minutes a day) can improve the quality of your sleep by 65%.

There are many ways to get the sleep-enhancing exercise your body needs. Walking is one just about anyone can do. Maybe you've already tried that. Maybe you're looking for something new. What are the most effective types of exercise for a better night's sleep? Which one suits you and your lifestyle best?

Here, the most effective way is to do moderate exercise. Find a way of getting moving during the day in order to improve the quality of sleep, as working out the entire body and mind can enable you to sleep soundly. Research suggests that moderate aerobic exercise can help boost the quality of sleep as well as the time you take to fall asleep. Only do exercise in moderation as doing vigorous exercise has not shown to boost the sleep patterns. You realize that regular aerobic exercises like walking cannot guarantee to cure insomnia but can offer good benefits to sleep patterns.

On the other hand, don't do exercise 3 hours before bedtime since exercise activates your cells and keep you awake.

Actually, the alertness impact caused by exercise can last up to 3 hours, and can reduce the amount of melatonin. Though this hormone facilitates you to sleep, it's recommended to exercise first thing after waking up. Doing so can help wake up and rev your metabolism in order to boost your energy the entire day. If you can't yet decide what you can do, these exercises can be done at any location without having to strain a lot:

Exercise 1

-Position your back against a wall and then lower until the upper legs are parallel to the ground.

-Then shuffle the feet until the lower legs become parallel to the wall that's behind you. Ensure that the knees are bent to 90 degrees.

-Now hold the arm in front of you and stay in this position for about 10-30 seconds. Repeat these exercises for about 2-3 times.

Exercise 2

-Position a chair next to a firm place like a wall or cubicle. Then turn your chair 45 degrees to the right

-Extend the left arm straight out to the side at your shoulder height and then push against this surface.

-Keep the back of the palm against this surface and then repeat the exercises on the right side.

-Do the exercises for around 5-6 times.

Exercise 3

-Position the hands on the wall shoulder width apart

-Then lean on the wall and start to push as hard as possible

-Continue to push with the same strength for around 15 seconds. Relax and repeat as desired.

Dance

Getting down is one of the ways to relieve tense muscles and fight stress, as it gets the body moving and curbs muscular pains and aches. When you dance, blood is pumped into the vessels and your heart starts racing. Hormones and endorphins are also released and thus you feel energized and able to sleep soundly. A light dance should help you experience fun and forget all the stress and anxiety in life especially when accompanied with some fast-paced music to make it a joyous experience.

Though all dances can greatly relieve stress, fast paced dances are the best among them tango, hip-hop, swing and salsa. If you have a partner, you can attend a dancing class to help both of you to do the dance as a joint activity. To begin dancing, start slow, get a few songs you enjoy; or songs that can let you follow the tempo.

-Be in a comfortable outfit in order to allow you to bend or sway to the muscle easily. Look for ample space free from obstruction

-If possible, dim the lights and shelf all problems you have. Only pay attention to the music, think calm, and cleanse your thoughts.

-Stretch with your arms and slow bending poses in order to relieve stress, as you move slowly to the music.

-Take a number of deep breaths, smile, and shelf all worries, maintain the balance, and move in time to your music.

-Then change to fast-paced music. Shift to a strong, loud and refreshing music and dance to it as if your life depends on it! Allow all stress, anger, and anxiety to escape until you feel energized. By now, your focus should be on the dancing, not the problems.

-Gradually slow down in order to calm down and avoid possible exhaustion. Once relaxed, take a healthy drink or some water and continue listening to soft music.

- Create a playlist that consists of nature sounds such as birds chirping, bubbling brook, or the ocean. Then let the mind focus on the variety of instruments, melodies or singers in one piece.

-Alternatively, you can blow off steam by rocking out to more upbeat tunes, or maybe sing at the top of the lungs.

Walk

Walking is a very effective way to relieve stress as it puts your mind in a meditative mood, especially when walking in a green area or park. This practice helps boost the production of endorphins that reduce stress, as well as increased energy levels and less fatigue. Walking should help you fight stress and sleeplessness and strengthen your heart.

On top of improved sleep, another benefit is that walking helps to lose weight, feel lighter and allow you to exercise more. This is because you burn calories and increase muscle tone and mass and also boost the rate of metabolism. Walking is also important because it exposes you to natural sunlight, which boosts vitamin D in your body. Vitamin D plays a major role in the body like improving the bone health and immunity.

Here are a few tips to use when walking to reduce stress that interferes with restful sleep:

-Focus on your senses while outside in order to forget about the anxious thoughts. For instance, what are the smells, sights, or sounds of nature?

-Walk in a quiet place such as around a lake or a park.

-Do not rush; just take it easy, making your strides as short as possible.

-Take some deep breaths to relieve tension from your head down to your feet.

Yoga

Here's something I'll bet you didn't know. In the human nervous system, sleep onset and yoga are closely related. Specifically, the parasympathetic nervous system (which governs digestion and relaxation) is where yoga and sleep converge.

Dr. L. G. Khalsa, at the Division of Sleep Medicine (Brigham and Women's Hospital, Harvard University), has conducted a study that reveals the profound impact yoga can have on human sleep patterns. The study's results showed that the full spectrum of the various yoga styles in the discipline improved sleep duration, and reduced the time it took for participants in the study to fall asleep.

Yoga can help you change your lifestyle and reduce stress through mindfulness, a practice that can increase your awareness of the unity of body and mind. Mindfulness also boosts unity of the unconscious thoughts, behaviors, and feelings and thus may undermine your spiritual, physical, and emotional health. The mind is prone to stress and other stress-related disorders, in which mindfulness has resulted into a positive outcome. Being mindful can help reduce your emotional reactivity, overall arousal, and lower blood pressure.

Yoga can easily be incorporated with mindfulness to help change sedentary lifestyle even in people with stress related hormonal problems. Yogis can learn on how to make informed choices and follow techniques aimed at improving their own health. This lifestyle coaching can include various aspects like stress reduction, exercising, diet, mindfulness, and other relaxation techniques.

What you need to do is try out specific yoga poses that are designed for relaxation. These poses are designed to make your body relax, to eliminate fatigue and to make the body feel lighter. Relaxation poses are known to lower high blood pressure, monitor the respiratory system and to induce high quality sleep. The poses also help cure mental imbalance, lack of memory, insomnia, heart disease and other conditions. They make you feel calmer, alert, and energetic in your entire day.

But before trying out yoga exercises, observe the following:

- Ensure you are physically fit and free from possible medical issues that may trigger serious heart or blood pressure problems. Talking to a health practitioner is a good consideration.

- Seek for an environment that is of low-pressure, to allow you work at your own pace. When stretching, ensure you don't overdo it beyond your ability.

- Dress comfortably, in an outfit that can allow full range of motion. As yoga is best done on bare feet, look for shoes that you can slip on and off easily.

- The easiest method is to learn yoga from a DVD, an instructional book or from a website. However, you can find a yoga class or an instructor. To get yoga classes, visit your local gyms, yoga studios or YMCAs and community centers. You can also attend yoga colleges or hire a private instructor.

Once done with the precautions you can then try out these 8 easy poses to make everything under control:

- **Easy pose**

The poses are designed to make a person comfortable, where you sit cross-legged comfortably on the carpet or ground. You need to be in a meditation pose though not for long time as a beginner. Follow these steps:

-Sit on the carpet or yoga mat in a comfortable position

-Then bend both knees and be at a cross-legged position with your waist, back and neck being in a straight line.

-Ensure that the hands are on your knees. Fix the index finger with the tip of the thumb, with the other three fingers straight.

-Continue to breathe rhythmically

The pose is designed for meditation and can be practiced as long as you can bear. Gently increase your duration of practice to 15 or 30 minutes. It's advisable to have a cushion to support your bottom, and to help you sit straight and for longer. When free or relaxed, set some time to practice seated in asana as opposed to sitting on chair or sofa.

Easy Pose
Sukhasana

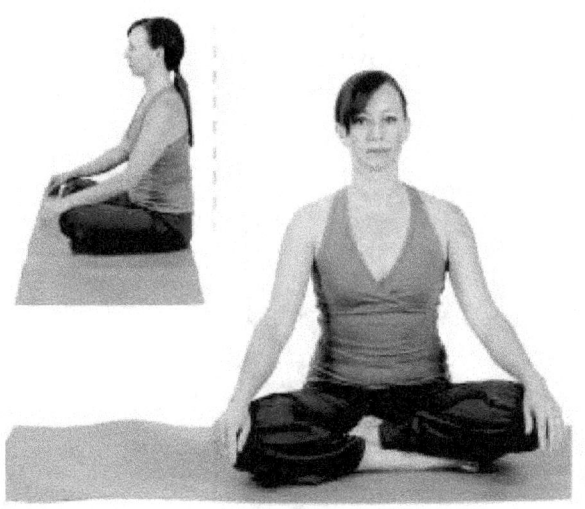

- **Seated Pose**

This pose can be easiest for you as you do it in a sitting position. The pose is meant to facilitate blood circulation to body organs and muscles being exercised. Your body will be relaxed and the breath harmonized, which will ultimately allow you to sleep for longer. To practice this:

- Sit on your carpet or yoga mat and then spread both your legs forward, with both legs resting on the carpet.

-Maintain the legs straight, ensuring that you don't bend the legs at your knee joint

-Sit with your upper half of the body reclined backwards slightly, with both hands on the carpet for support. The palms should be downwards and the fingers to the rear.

-Now keep the arms and back straight

-Then turn the head erect or gently tilt it towards either of your shoulder. Continue to breathe as usual paying attention to your breath and experience your body getting relaxed.

-Do this relaxation pose after each pose to ensure you are relaxed while sitting. As a beginner, you may need to rest after every pose; though with practice you'll rest after around 3-4 poses. However, the main objective is to relax to an extent of obtaining sleep so you don't have to sweat yourself into exhaustion!

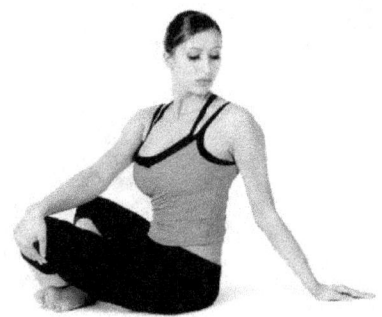

- **Corpse Pose**

Here you don't have to kill yourself in order to turn into a dead body but rather try to assume the copse posture for relaxation. You will relax your entire limbs and soon you will get into dreamland. Let's see how you do it:

-Lie down in a supine position, on a carpet, mat or other comfortable surface

-Keep your legs apart about 1-1 ½ feet from each other

-Put both hands further away from the side of your body

-Then allow the left toe point towards the left with the right toe facing towards the right

-You can keep the head either straight or inclined towards the right or left

-Ensure that your palm is facing upward, and the whole body is in a straight line and fully relaxed

-Now gently close your eyes

-Start to imagine that your entire body is relaxed; to facilitate relaxation of each body organ. Pay attention on entire body parts from the head to toe and experience your body becoming lighter.

-While in this pose, practice your normal rhythmic breathing.

- Once fully relaxed, don't get up with a jerk; but open the eyes gradually and then get up slowly

The pose is meant to give the rest of your body relaxation, and can be carried out at the end of daily yoga routine. When fatigued to do any other pose, practice the pose for relaxation and progress to other poses. However, ensure that you eliminate tension from your mind and fight thoughts that trigger stress in order to be relaxed. To your surprise, you might not even complete the pose and may soon fall asleep! People who regularly practice copse pose claim it induces sleep.

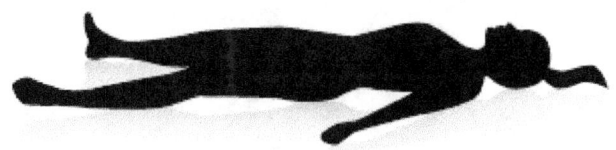

- **Lotus Pose**

The pose is recommendable for yoga breathing poses and meditation as its practice results into peace of mind. Try to:

-Sit on the carpet or yoga mat with legs spread forwards

-Now bend your right knee at the knee joint, and hold the right foot using both of your hands. You should hold the ankle of your right leg using the right hand and then catch the toes of the right leg using the left hand.

-Then lift the right foot upwards and then position it on the right thigh, to ensure that the right heel is very close to the navel.

-Bend the knee of the left leg and hold your left foot using both hands. You should hold the ankle of the left leg and then catch the toes of the left leg with the right hand.

-Then lift the left foot and fix the left heel at the base of your right thigh.

-Ensure that both knees are on the ground with the soles of the feet pointing upward. However, you can switch the position of your legs after getting uncomfortable

-Keep your neck and back straight, with both eyes closed.

-Maintain the hands on the knees, touching the index finger with the tip of the thumb; while the other 3 fingers remain straight.

When starting with this pose, do it for 30 seconds and then prolong the duration, as you get comfortable with the asana.

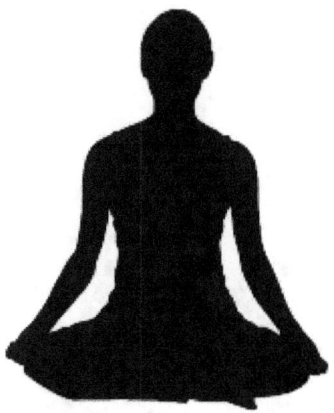

- The Locust pose

Don't confuse this with the lotus pose above! This pose is important to relieve stress, and can help you relax and get some sleep.

-Lie down on your belly with the face looking down, and the chin resting gently on the floor.

-Place the legs together, and then stretch the leg back with the toes stretching outward.

-Ensure that the pubis is firmly pressed into the mat, and maintain the arms stretched back with the palms up. Be as relaxed as possible.

-Clench the hands to form fists, and then stiffen the arms, legs, and knees.

-Breathe in slowly, in order to exert a little pressure on the balled fists; and lift the legs together as high as possible. Do not bend the legs.

-Try to hold the pose for 15-30 seconds while you hold your breath as long as you can bear.

-Then breathe out slowly as you lower your legs gently.

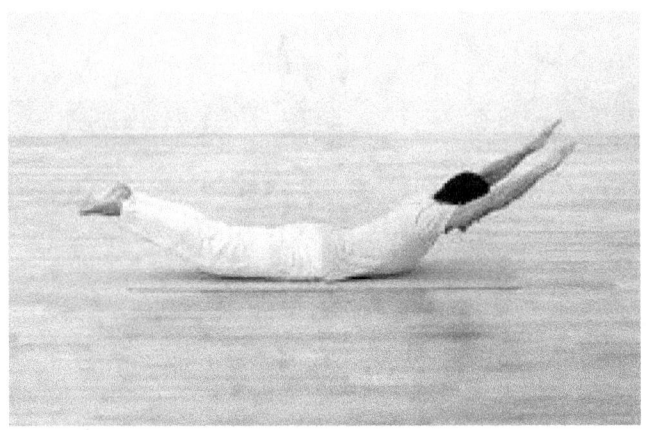

- **Half spinal twist**

The asana should help boost the capacity of lungs in order for it to handle more oxygen. Follow these steps:

-With legs stretched out straight in front of you, sit up while you keep the feet together and the spike upright.

-Bend the left leg and position the heel of the left feet beside the right hip or rather maintain the left leg straight.

-Then take the right leg over the left knee and put the left hand onto the right knee, the right hand being behind you.

-Now twist at the waist, shoulders and neck in this pattern to the right and look over your right shoulder. Hold and progress with gentle long breaths in and out.

-Return to the initial pose, exhale, and then release the right hand that is behind you. Then release the waist, the chest, and finally the neck, and sit up straight. Repeat on your other side.

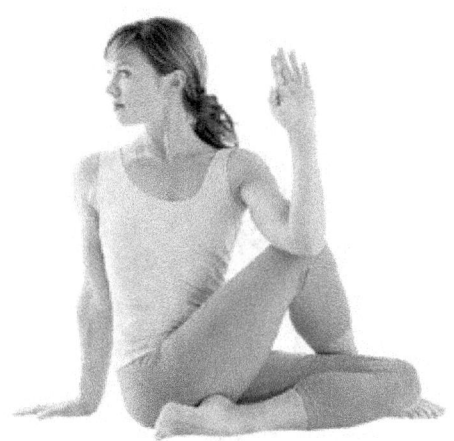

- **Tree pose**

-Stand with feet together and then shift most of the weight to one leg.

-Raise the leg with the little weight in order for the foot to face inwards, to the direction of the opposite knee. To help you pull up the leg, hold your ankle.

-Put the heel of the foot onto the inner thigh of the leg on the ground, very close to the pelvis as you can.

-Then raise the hands gently above the head while fingers point to the ceiling. Focus your mind and control your balance.

To maintain the pose and avoid falling over, ensure that you stare at one spot in front of you and breathe steadily. Do not support on the wall or chair as this reduces the intensity of the tree pose.

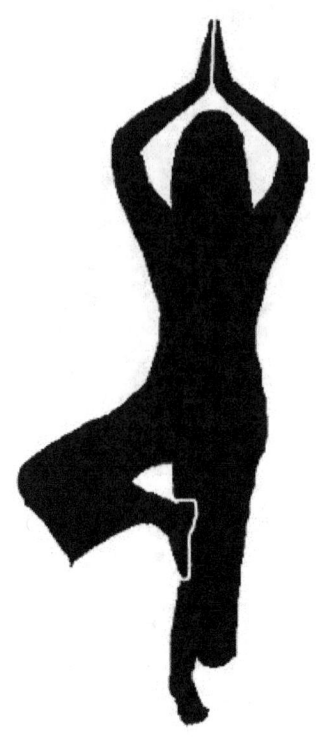

- **Half moon pose**

Follow these steps:

-Begin by standing with your feet together. Then raise hands over the head and now clasp the palms together. You should extend your stretch by attempting to reach the ceiling.

-Breathe out and then gradually bend sideways from the hips, as you keep the hands together. Keep the elbows straight without bending forward; and appreciate the stretch feeling from the fingertips and thighs.

-Breathe in and return to standing pose. Repeat the half-moon pose on the other side.

Yoga may involve more of a time commitment, but its proven efficacy is worth a look. See the Resources section at the end of this book for more information. You may find that yoga is the silver bullet to a good night's sleep for you.

Swimming

Who doesn't like a nice swim? You don't have to be Michael Phelps to make it count, either. Being in the water and moving around takes more effort than you think, as it's the resistance of the water against your body, as well as moving in a different element that's at the heart of swimming's health benefits. Researchers have found that swimming increases sleep quality by 50%, so it's worth investigating, if you're feeling sleep-deprived.

Most of us don't have access to our own, personal swimming facilities, so finding out where your local community center is will get you started. If the community center doesn't have a pool, try the local YMCA/YWCA, or health club. Many of these facilities offer affordable pool access and even swimming and Aquafit classes. These days, you can even take a water pole dancing class, so you can have a ball and sleep better while you're at it! Find more information about Aquafit and water pole dancing in the Resources section.

Geo-caching

Geo-caching is a great activity on many levels. For one, it's an outdoor pursuit and there's nothing like fresh air to help you sleep better. For another, it's something you can do with family and friends and also, it's a way to meet new people. Finally, it's something that adds value to your life by engaging you in something that takes you out of yourself and your daily concerns. It's both exercise and an absorbing hobby.

Think "treasure hunt" to understand the point of geo-caching. Using GPS devices, participants locate logbooks secured in outdoor locations, inside waterproof containers. From these log books, they follow clues to find a variety of objects hidden in the area.

Geo-caching is now a global phenomenon, involving millions

of people in locations all over the world. See the Resources section to find out where you can connect with geo-caching in your area.

Cycling

You don't have to ride far and you don't even have to risk life and limb on the roads, anymore, to enjoy and benefit from cycling. Most large cities and many towns now boast bike lanes. Helmet up and keep your wits about you and you'll find that cycling is a healthy, outdoor exercise option that can put you on the road to sleeping well.

Cycling needn't break the bank, either. It's possible to find bicycles in good working order at local second hand shops. Volunteers will often repair these bikes to get them road ready and suitable for resale. Add an effective lock and a desire to see your surroundings from the perspective of a bicycle and you have ignition!

Breathe in. Breathe out

Now that you have carved out a little extra time from your day and you've begun to experience the benefits of taking control of the little things, you can take a breath.

Quite literally.

Breathing is something we do without thinking. With one inhalation (a breath in) and one exhalation (a breath out) combining as a respiration, the average person breathes between 20,000 and 25,000 times each day. Dr. Andrew Weil believes that the simple act of breathing in and out can be employed as an effective sleep aid.

Dr. Weil's medical training focused on holistic practices. Part of this focus was the study of breathing and how it can be used to treat a variety of ailments, including disordered sleep patterns. Dr. Weil's contention is that deep breathing, following a pattern prescribed by the ancient practice of pranayama, can send us to sleep in as little as 60 seconds.

Hard to believe? Not so fast!

The "4-7-8" pattern works for a number of reasons. Principle among these is that the deep breaths prescribed work to expel carbon dioxide from the body. This profound breathing also works to tranquilize the central nervous system. The technique, if practiced regularly, will also ease anxiety and tension. Less of these in your life is yet another way to rest better.

To enhance both the physical and mental wellbeing and to keep chronic stress monitored, practice this 3-minute exercise at any time. The breathing exercise can help you decrease feelings of anger, frustration, or tension.

-Sit comfortably at an upright posture

-Pay attention to your current state and existence, and block those intrusive thoughts that creep up. Keep the eyes closed as well.

-Now concentrate on how you breathe. Start inhaling through the nose, take a few seconds.

-Then exhale through the mouth, and attempt to make the exhalation last 2 times longer than inhalation.

-Progress with the breathing technique for 3-5 minutes. If you enjoy the alertness and relieved state of mind, increase the practice session to around 15-20 minutes daily.

-Continue to exercise regularly in order to achieve relaxation in stressful conditions.

Once done with the breathing exercise, slowly progress into muscular relaxation exercise for complete relief. There are other breathing exercises that you can also try out:

- **Exercise 1**

-Look for a quiet and calm place and relax for about 15-20 minutes. The best pose would be sitting with the back straight, but try your own method. When you inhale, do so through the stomach and then the chest, but first ensure you don't have a heart problem.

-Soften a little up, and choose a comfortable pose, either standing or sitting. Relax your hands and try softening the knees. Then drop the shoulders and finally relax your jaws.

-Begin to breathe in gradually through your nose, starting from a count of 4. Maintain the shoulders down, while the stomach expands as you inhale. If possible, attempt to hold your breath for 5-10 seconds.

-Now release the breath gradually and quite smoothly, through a count of 7. Once done, repeat the entire exercise for around 10-15 minutes.

- **Exercise 2**

-Relax your shoulders and close your throat slightly. At this position, ensure that you can hear your breath as you breathe in.

-Using your thumbs, cover the ears and the eyes using the fingers. Keep the lips lightly closed and the teeth being slightly apart. Relax the jaws and then exhale. Ensure that you make a continuous humming sound. Ensure that your relaxation is long and smooth.

-Repeat this exercise about 5-10 and then sit. Then do some long and slow breaths for a few minutes. Enjoy the peace of mind and wait to fall asleep.

- **Exercise 3**

1. Place one hand on your belt-line, and then other one over the chest, just on top of your breastbone. You should easily feel the part of your body or the muscles used in breathing.

2. Open the mouth and then let out a gentle sigh, allowing your shoulders and your body muscles to relax, down as you exhale. The sigh is meant to relax your upper body muscles, but not to fully empty your lungs.

3. Now keep your mouth closed and then pause for about 15 seconds. With the mouth closed, inhale slowly through the nose, ensuring that you push your stomach outwards as you breathe. Your belly movement should slightly precede your inhalation as this breathing motion is pulling the air in.

4. Inhale as much air as possible, and ensure not to throw your upper body into it. When done, now stop with the inhalation exercise.

5. Pause for as long as you can, depending on your comfort or lung size. Remember that as you breathe through this technique, you are inhaling larger portions of air and therefore you should breathe more gradually as you normally do. Taking shallow and small breaths can result into lightheadedness that may result into yawning. In case you feel lightheaded, just slow down, as this is just normal.

6. Open your mouth, and then slowly exhale through your mouth. As you breathe out, pull your belly in. Now pause and continue practicing step 3-6.

7. Continue to practice the breathing exercises for a few more minutes. To ensure that you're breathing correctly, use your hands to detect where there is muscular movement of the breathing.

The breathing movement should occur at your stomach, and thus your upper body should remain quite still. In case you notice your head and shoulders moving upwards or feel the movement on the chest, you should start at step 1. This will ensure that the motion is made at your stomach.

- Measure the breath

This is a different technique of deep breathing that can also help you relax and fall asleep peacefully. Here's how you do it:

1. Soften a little up, and then choose to either sit or stand. Ensure you relax your hands and soften your knees. Now drop your shoulders and then allow your jaw to relax.

2. At this position, breathe in slowly through the nose. Start to count from 1-4, and keep your shoulders down. Ensure that your stomach can expend as you breathe in. Try to hold your breath for a few seconds.

3. When done, slowly release your breath very smoothly, as you do a count of 1-7. Repeat this technique for about 10-15 minutes.

- **Breathe like The Bumble Bee**

This is quite a fun-activity that you can practice when alone in the house. As the name suggests, this technique involves making some noise to calm your mind and de-clutter the mind. To practice this bubble bee breathing exercise:

1. Start by relaxing your shoulders and then close your throat slightly. You should be in a position to hear your breath as you inhale air.

2. With your thumbs, cover your ears and use your fingers to cover your eyes. Maintain your lips lightly closed with the teeth slightly apart and your jaws should be relaxed. Now breathe out slowly ensuring to make long and a humming sound. Your relaxation should be long and very smooth.

3. Repeat this technique about 5-10 times and then sit. Do some long and slow breaths for a few minutes. Enjoy the peace.

- **Abdominal Breathing**

-Place one hand on the chest and the other on the belly, and then take a deep breath through your nose. When doing so, make sure it's only the diaphragm that inflates but not your chest; fill it with air to create a stretch into your lungs.

-Then take 6-10 slow but deep breaths every minute for a period of 15 minutes daily in order to improve your mental clarity and fight anxiety. Continue with the exercises for 6-8 weeks or longer if desired.

The technique is very effective for occasional sleeplessness, though people who experience persistent stress might find it harder to control breath.

- **Alternate Nostril Breathing**

This technique is known to bring calm and balance, and to unite the left and right sides of your brain. It works best in crunch time, or when you need to focus or gain energy.

-Start on a comfortable position; hold your right thumb over the right nostril as you breathe in deeply through the left nostril.

-As you reach the peak of inhaling, use the ring finger to close the left nostril and then breathe out through your right nostril.

-Continue with this pattern; breathe in through the right nostril and using the right thumb to close it off. Finally exhale through your left nostril.

- **Skull Shining Breath**

This exercise starts from a long and slow inhale that is followed by a fast and strong exhale from your lower belly.

-Begin at a comfortable pose and start breathing in and out. Then pace up to one inhale-exhale through your nose for each 1-2 seconds. Perform these exercises for about 10 breaths.

-The technique is applicable after you wake up, and can help warm up your body and eliminate the stale energy, therefore waking up the brain. The exercise is abdominal intensive and is best done after a shot of coffee.

Once done with these exercises, you can peacefully rest and get lost into the dreamland! Please see the link to Dr. Weil's demonstration of the 4-7-8 techniques in the Resources section.

Visualize

Our minds are always filled with countless thoughts, worries, and other forms of mental clutter that makes it hard for us to even notice the things that are happening at the moment. This preoccupation of our minds makes us stressed, sleepless and depressed because we don't stop for any moment to just be in the moment. However, you can try to visualize being at a different relaxing setting even without moving an inch! As a way to get mindful, get lost into your world of imagination to help ease troubled mind. You can:

1. Think of a calming experience

Visualize yourself viewing something quite calming such as a pool of water, waterfall, or a green field under a rainbow. Then see yourself venturing into relaxing activities such as smelling roses, floating down the river, staring at the blue sky on a perfect day, gliding over clouds or any other activity that describes your ideal fantasy. Try to explore your place of fantasy, and appreciate every aspect of this imaginary realm.

2. Try story telling

A good way to calm down is to share stories with workmates, kids or other people. You can create a storyline every evening, based on a light and happy state of mind. For instance, think about an interesting movie scene and then visualize acting a few episodes say those of daring rescue.

3. Visualize doing an activity that both you and your partner enjoy doing. For instance, imagine your lover, boyfriend, girlfriend or spouse walking beside you through a field of flowers that has calming aroma.

4. Construct your imaginary house or room in your mind. Find out what scenery or design you admire most and try building a magnificent architecture. What colors would you go for? Ensure that you're entirely lost into your dreams and that this distraction helps you relax.

5. Also imagine the ideal sleeping environment for you, such as being curled up with your dream partner on a soft cloud, sleeping under the stars or being curled up on a feather-bed that has the softest sheets.

6. Imagine that you see a swinging pendulum. Close your eyes get relaxed and then experience the sensation of having to "fall into the mattress"

7. Start to imagine of those impossible or strange activities such as chasing after bankers, growing red wings that has dangling yellow fishhooks or walking on walls like a 'superman" etc.

In order to get into actual visualization, try these steps:

-Sit in a comfortable posture, eyes closed and then take a few deep breaths starting from the diaphragm. Make sure that you relax the muscles in your stomach.

-Start to imagine that you are witnessing a beautiful scenery that is full of radiant white light. At this point, experience the light that fills you with bliss and serenity

-Now inhale the radiant white light while allowing the light to be fully absorbed into your body with every breath that you take. Allow this radiant light to reach your organs and wash every cell and atom in the body. Ensure that you become fully absorbed in the light.

-Then visualize yourself as exhaling the sleep-disturbing thoughts, which escape from you as a thick black smoke. Also try to get your stable state of mind and then shift on the current feeling after achieving it. Progress to inhale the image of the good feeling with each breath you take.

-Try to imagine a very real or detailed visual image, which should incorporate all aspects of color, smell, feelings, and sound. To achieve this experience, try the following sensory based imaginations:

- For color or beautiful sight, venture into an art museum, or wander around a well-kept neighborhood or garden. Also obtain those beautiful pictures from a textbook you enjoy reading.

- For sound, include some relaxing music. You can also choose scenery where there are birds singing, wind rustling through tress or waves that crash upon a beach.

- For smell, include a few scented candles or try smelling favorite flowers in a garden. Try your deodorant or perfume, or stop by a bakery if possible. If in your office, just breathe in the clean and fresh air.

- For taste, you can enjoy some delicious cup of tea or coffee. If hungry, prepare a nice meal and then eat it slowly. Ensure you appreciate and enjoy every bite.

- For a sense of touch, take a warm bubble bath, or instead wrap yourself in a soft blanket. You can also get a massage, pet your cat, or dog or alternatively sit outside in the cool breeze.

Reading

Once you're done with a few demanding tasks, commit yourself to reading a book as a way to calm the racing thoughts. You can read any article, but try a calming book that gets you nodding off. Reading under natural light is recommendable since artificial light can cause sleeplessness; and can work in a similar manner as meditation.

On the other hand, reserve few minutes after 6PM to do breathing techniques in order to be relaxed enough and less tired. You can practice anywhere, though you may choose to lie on the carpet or bed for comfort. Begin to breathe in gently and watch the stomach rise, in a bid to inhale and exhale 6 times per minute.

-Inhale deeply for 4-6 long counts, and then hold your breath for a count of 4.

-Continue to take deep breaths for 4 counts, and then push the last breath gently.

-Repeat the exercise. Ensure that you pay attention to your breath, and remain focused on it.

Meditate

Meditation is the practice of getting your mind to start being in the moment and to tame those random thoughts that make you miss some of the most beautiful moments because you were overly obsessed about the future or the past. There are different ways of practicing mindfulness meditation, from mindful yoga, sounds and thoughts mediation, and silent meditation with bells. The following guide should help you practice most common forms of meditations and almost everywhere.

1. Choose a relaxed place

Locate a peaceful spot where there isn't any distraction or clutter, either indoors or outdoors. If preferred, you can leave the lights on or alternatively meditate on natural light. In order to fully calm and relax your mind, ensure you are in comfortable clothing, and without any shoes. You may choose to wear a sweater if doing meditation outdoors to avoid cold since extreme cold may cause distractions. You should also try to open the collar of your shirt or blouse, and remove your belt just to ensure that you are comfortable.

2. Decide practice duration

Decide the amount of time you want to mediate, up to 45 minutes or an hour. You may have two sessions both in the morning or evening, or a single session if very busy. You can try silent mediation exercise that is interspersed with gentle bells at 5, 10, 15, 20 and 30 minutes to determine time. Such an approach is good in boosting your confident as well as helping you to pace yourself. Gradually, you can learn meditation sessions without requiring any guidance.

3. Take a posture

There are various ways of taking a good posture, such as sitting on a meditation cushion a chair, the floor, or a park bench,; as far as it's solid and stable. If sitting on a cushion on the floor, cross legs in front of you. Likewise, if on a chair or a bench, the bottoms of your feet should touch the floor.

Straighten your body but do not stiffen and then position your upper arms parallel to the upper body. Then allow the hands to drop into the top of your legs. Drop the chin a little and let your gaze to fall down gently. You may let your eyelids lower and let whatever that appears before your eyes remain there without focusing on it. Be in this posture for a few moments and follow the next breath that comes out.

4. Concentrate

Though you meditate for the purpose of falling asleep, being in the moment both in your mind and body is an important part of meditation. You need to focus in a bid to keep off distractions that could easily make it hard for you to achieve the state of pure consciousness. Failure to realize the calming benefits of mediation may not facilitate sleep and would be a total let-down. To help you get more concentration, you should:

- Close your eyes

Though meditation may be done with both eyes closed or opened, you may need to close the eyes to block the external and virtual stimuli or other distractions. Once you're accustomed to regular meditation, you may try meditating while your eyes are open. This may be helpful if you find concentrating with eyes closed difficult. When you open your eyes, ensure you don't focus on other objects, or get easily distracted.

- Focus on a visual object

You can think of constructive mental images such as imagining of a lotus flower that sits in your belly rising and falling with your breath or a buoy floating in the ocean and moving up and down with your breathing patterns. When your mind seems to wander, try to refocus on the breathing technique without thinking of anything else.

To enhance your concentration, you can focus on your breathing, a mantra, a specific object, or an image. You can for instance observe the flame of a burning candle or a hole and anything else that makes you keep off distractions. This form of open-eye meditation is especially easy if you have something to focus on. Other objects that you can choose from include flowers, crystals, statues, or pictures of divine beings.

Position the image at your eye level to ensure that you don't strain your head while focusing on it. Now gaze on it without getting distracted, up to when your peripheral vision begins to dim, and the object takes over your vision. After being entirely focused without any response to other stimuli, you should experience a refreshing sense of profound serenity. After you're ready for actual meditation; you can then try out the following meditation techniques:

5-Minute Meditation

As meditation works better when done regularly, you can do a daily meditation program of 5 minutes to relieve stress and bring happiness. Learn how you can utilize your 5 minutes here:

-Get a timer such as an alarm clock, a 5-minute music, a mobile phone, or any other device, and set for 5 minutes. Relax, close your eyes, and take a few breaths from your diaphragm, to release tension from the body.

-Keep your mind free from thoughts but instead focus on your 'being' rather than thinking on nothing. When other thoughts come into your mind, just ignore them and get back to your present moment.

-Continue with this practice for 5 minutes, for better relaxation and improved sleep. You should carry out this practice regularly.

Bath Meditation

You can try this technique to obtain the benefits arising from a relaxing and soothing hot bath that allows stress to be released from your muscles. Once you're relaxed, you're able to obtain a restful sleep as you may require. To make such a bath meditation set-up, refer to this guideline:

-Make time for meditation, such as 15 minutes of uninterrupted practice. Buy a few aromatherapy bathing products such as peppermint or lavender scented soap to make stress relief more effective.

-Get into the bath water and relax. Allow your breathing to be deeper and slower, allow your belly to rise and fall naturally with the breathing patterns.

-Pay your attention to the sensations that come from your body, such as the warmth of the water on your skin or the pressure the tub exerts on your back. Release your thoughts, keep your mind calm as you try to focus as much as possible to the present moment.

-Continue with the bath meditation, for a few minutes, until you feel soothed and well relaxed. Ensure that thoughts of the past or internal dialogue do not affect your concentration.

Meditate With Aromatherapy

Aromatherapy is a way of utilizing the natural oils extracted from plants to improve the physical and psychological well-being. As a form of therapy, you stand to benefit from a relaxed mind, body, and soul. Even if you are new to meditation, you can easily create an easy aromatherapy session. Follow this guideline:

-Adopt a relaxed posture and then light a stick of incense such as lavender stick incense, following the package directions

-Wait for trails of smoke to curl and waft upwards and then

watch the smoke. Just allow your mind to be immersed in the various patterns or paths that the smoke trails take.

-Do not allow other thoughts to come into your mind, by trying to bring your attention to the trails coming from the incense. Wait for a moment, and appreciate the elegant and simple display.

-You can inhale the refreshing aroma as much as possible, based on your ability to focus. To start with, you can try 5-10 minutes a number of times per week, and later try daily for a longer duration of 30 minutes.

-Try lavender, peppermint, and sage scents but be careful not to have the smoke trails too close to your eyes or nose. If you have respiratory problem with burning incense, you may do other meditation practices instead.

Loving Kindness Meditation

You find this funny, huh? This technique forms one of the popular practices and focuses on loving energy towards your mind. This practice is important in making you experience the warm feelings of loving kindness, on top of regular benefits of meditation. You can follow this simple technique for happiness, to fight stress and sleeplessness. The technique can consume a hell of a time thus practice it when you experience extended periods of sleeplessness. Follow these steps:

-Locate a silent or relaxing place and sit in your most comfortable posture. Keep your eyes closed, muscles relaxed and then take slow and deep breaths.

-Imagine that you are witnessing a perfect emotional or physical wellness or inner peace. Also imagine that you are experiencing complete love, you are thankful to yourself for everything you are. Acknowledge that you are right, in whatever state you are.

-Make 3-4 repetition of positive reassuring phrases to yourself; any mantra that you find relaxing. You can adopt phrases such as "May I be happy" or "peaceful sleep". If it's already at night, you don't have to make unnecessary noise. You can recite the mantra silently to yourself.

-Bask in this experience for some time, redirecting your feelings back to your mantra in case your mind seems to wander. Try to receive as much benefits from these feelings of loving or kindness.

-Based on your preference, you may choose to stay in this kind of meditation, or shift your focus to those people that you treasure. Begin with a close friend or a relative, and try to feel your love or gratitude for them. You may decide to repeat your phrase that contributes to feelings of loving kindness within you.

-After holding these positive feelings towards a person, now extend the loving kindnesses to other important people from your life into your consciousness.

-Examine these people one by one, and then envision them with the same perfect wellness and inner peace.

-From here, you can further extend to another group of people such as neighbors, acquaintances or other people you share similar ideas. These may include people you are often in a conflict so that you can find ways of greater peace or forgiveness.

-After you are done with meditation, open your eyes and then acknowledge the possibility of revisiting that wonderful feeling in your entire day. You can memorize the feelings of loving kindness, and then revisit the feeling through deep breaths and focus shift in a certain entire day.

The best way to start this meditation practice is from you as the subject before extending to other people. Though directing the meditation to troublesome people may allow room for forgiveness, it takes a lot patience to achieve this. To help control time you spend during meditation, you may set a timer starting with 5 minutes session.

Dear Diary

Did you ever keep a diary when you were a kid? Did you rush to it when you arrived home from school just itching to write the name of your secret crush of the moment in its pages? The thrill of putting that tiny key in that tiny lock was one of the greatest joys of my childhood.

Keeping a diary taught me a lot about what and who mattered to me and why. In the pages of my diary, I wrestled with the petty squabbles of childhood. In fact, I probably learned the meaning of the word "petty" by leafing through previous entries and being horrified by the fact I hadn't spoken to this friend or that for a week over absolutely nothing. Or a boy. (It was usually a boy).

Keeping a diary as an adult ("journaling" being the all-grown-up name for it) serves a similar function. Writing down what strikes us as important about the day's events is a way for us to pinpoint stresses in our lives. It's also a way to identify triggers that can set off anxiety and in turn, lack of sleep.

You needn't write an epic novel in a journal. You needn't even write. You can draw, doodle, and write quotes that inspire you, or use it as a scrapbook. The important thing is that you set aside a little of that time you've taken back from your busyness to do it. Journaling is a support for addressing things in your life you'd like to change or improve, or even just for re-booting at the end of the day and concluding it with something positive.

A Gift for You

Whatever you do, don't cheap out on the journal you're going to write in. Your journal should look like what it is – a special place where you spend dedicated time taking note of what's important to you and how you're growing as a person. It can also be a place where you mark your exercise progress. The improvements you'll be experiencing in your sleep can (and should) also be tracked here.

The effect should be the same as that experienced by children putting those little keys in those little locks on their secret diaries – the anticipation of creating something intended for no one but you.

Choose a journal as lavish as you can afford. Whether that's expressed in the quality of the paper or bindings, whatever you choose should be redolent of special purpose.

It's for you and you alone. Choose with that in mind.

A Nurturing Discipline

Choose the time of day you'll write in your journal every day. This is not something you can catch up on if you miss a day. That day and its events and the revelations they hold for you are gone, once they're gone. Stick to your journaling time as strictly as you can. Choose a realistic time of day to set aside for this purpose and then stick to it. Right before you begin to prepare for sleep (see "Sleep Hygiene) is a great time for this.

Remember – this is not a chore. This is a nurturing discipline. Like all the other activities you're now using time that you've taken back to enjoy, this one is intended to feed you. And it will. The more you do it and the greater intentionality you approach it with, the greater the rewards will be.

Write Your Heart

This isn't a food diary. This isn't a telephone log. Use your journaling time to hone in on the events of the day that stand out for you. Before putting pen to paper, take a moment. Close your eyes. Use your new breathing technique to quiet yourself and to make space for your thoughts. Then write down whatever it was that struck you as important about the day. Even the negative events have a purpose. They're the events you'll learn the most from. Even if you're going to draw a picture, or place a bus ticket between the pages to remind you of someone you met on your commute home, you're making note of your day's events as though they mattered. They do.

What happens to you in the course of your day, regardless of whether these incidents and experiences are momentous or seemingly inconsequential, have an impact on you. By writing about them, you can also make sense of them. By making sense of them, you are given the opportunity to process them into meaning that can feed your understanding of the world around you. In understanding lies an important key to peace and wellbeing. And those are the qualities that can propel you toward the night's rest you need.

Chapter 5: Optimizing Your Bedroom For Its Role

Have you ever given the place you sleep the kind of careful, critical consideration it deserves? Have you ever looked around your sleeping space and asked yourself how you might make it more conducive to a good night's sleep?

Too often, in seeking the magic formula for restful sleep, the actual, physical location in which we do it is overlooked. This may be because we don't place nearly enough value on the importance of quality sleep. That's quite strange, considering we now know the damaging effects a lack of sleep can have on our health, our work and our relationships. We know that so many of us suffer from less than ideal rest and we feel its effects cascading through every area of our waking lives.

Let's talk about how we can make our sleep space a beloved retreat from the world we move through each day. Let's talk about making it a sanctuary of sleep.

Go, Little Glow Worm

Many of us use our bedrooms as multi-purpose areas. In the corner, there's an overflowing laundry basket. On the bedside table, an assortment of books, hand lotions, medications and other bits and pieces. Across from the place we lay our heads, there's almost invariably a television.

And that must be the first thing you remove from your sleep space.

The average American watches 35 hours of television each week. That's 5 hours per day. I not only think that's quite enough, I think it's too much. Does it really need to follow you into the bedroom? The short answer is "no", but why?

Is it really such a bad idea to watch TV in bed?

Dr. Mathias Basner, a sleep specialist at the University of Pennsylvania, says that television viewed in bed, or immediately before bedtime, can heavily impact how well we sleep. Dr. David Dinges, a colleague of Basner's and psychologist at the UofP, agrees. A chronic lack of sleep can be directly attributed to overstimulation in the evening, caused by television viewing.

We may believe we're "unwinding", but what we're really doing is stimulating our brains into a state which is not conducive to sleep. Not only that, the lure of the cathode ray tube can keep us awake longer than we should be at night, depriving us of needed sleep. We fall asleep in front of it, because our bodies have passed the point at which we should have listened to them and gone to sleep in our beds, with the lights out and the TV off!

But it's not just the television we need to banish from our bedrooms. Laptops and portable mobile devices need to be left outside the door before we lay down at night, too. Not only do we fiddle with them (which keeps us awake longer than we should be), we're exposed to the glow from their screens.

Exposure to intense, late night light disturbs our sleep patterns by inhibiting the production of the sleep hormone melatonin. It's not supposed to be there at night! The same can be said of ambient light in urban areas. It can keep us awake at night, by sending our brains the message that alertness is required, as it is *light* and not *dark*. So why make it worse by inviting it into our bedrooms?

The Reading Room

It's not your bedroom. Reading in bed, while a beloved practice of many, is another way to keep your brain working long after it should have gone into sleep mode. While not everyone is the same, the rule of thumb is simple – if you find yourself thinking, "I should go to sleep now, but this book is so great", and you do that regularly, then reading is something you should do elsewhere.

Just as you're creating a serene space to get the quality sleep you need in your bedroom, create a reading nook. Dress it up as lavishly as you can, with pillows and a colorful throw. A chaise longue, or overstuffed chair with an ottoman is ideal for this purpose. Stack your favorite books next to your new reading nook, creating a place to put your current reading material. Relax and enjoy.

Fido Doesn't Sleep Here Anymore

I know you love your furry friends. We all love them. But the bedroom is your sleeping space, not theirs. While this may sound pet-unfriendly and will no doubt set some animal-lovers off, Fido and Fluffy need to sleep elsewhere.

The Mayo Clinic Sleep Disorders Center's director, John Shephard, conducted a survey of some of his pet-owning patients. Of the sample surveyed, 60% permitted their pets to sleep with them. Incredibly, half this number reported reduced sleep quality due to their pets being in the bedroom.

And why do pets keep us up at night? Believe it nor not, many of them hog the bed. Why wouldn't they be? The message you're sending them is that your bed is theirs, too. Of course they think a rather huge patch of it belongs to them. Even worse, some pets snore (including our feline friends). My personal experience of sleeping with pets has been mixed, but overall, that experience has not been one of enhanced sleep. If you're seeking a better night's rest, then it's time to close the door.

Set up special, cushy sleeping arrangements for your pets to bed down in for the night. Trust me. They'll get over their initial surprise about the new arrangement, and be even happier to see you in the morning!

Blues, Stay Away from Me

We've already discussed some of the consequences of inviting the light from television, mobile devices and laptops into your sleeping sanctuary. We've also reviewed the effect of the modern, ever-illuminated night.

But did you know that the color of light could have a profound effect on your sleep quality, as well as your health?

All the types of electronics mentioned in this chapter emit blue light. This is highly beneficial to productivity and alertness during daylight hours. At night, though, exposure to it can have a serious effect on your sleep quality. Blue light is also found in lighting manufactured for optimum energy efficiency.

Researchers at Harvard University have found that blue light suppresses melatonin production (the hormone that helps you sleep) at twice the rate other types of light do.

While we all want to help the environment, LED and compact fluorescent lights should not be used in the bedroom. Instead, change your light bulbs to soft pink or red bulbs (perfect for nightlights). You're not reading in the bedroom anymore, so the reduced light won't be an issue and the change will contribute to a sound night's sleep.

The Zen of Sleep

Life's detritus follows us into our sleeping spaces. It collects there, creating chaos in what should be the most serene, calm area in our homes. I guess it's just what we're used to, but clutter and mess are another reason we can't sleep at night.

A new study, presented at the 2015 SLEEP conference, has found that hoarders have even more trouble sleeping than the average sleep-disturbed person. The chaos they live in the midst of is a red flag for all of us. Letting it all pile up, says Dr. Pamela Thacer, of St. Lawrence University, New York, is a recipe for sleep disaster. Dr. Thacer's study found a definitive link between clutter and sleeping disorders in a sample of 83 people at risk for being formally identified as hoarders. The control group (those who had little or no risk for hoarding disorder), showed higher sleep quality.

Look around your room. The worst offenders will be immediately identifiable. The first of these is likely laundry and clothing left on chairs or other surfaces where they shouldn't be. Pick it up, sort it out and then, resolve to hanging up those pieces of clothing you can wear again and putting the rest in the laundry basket.

Put the laundry basket somewhere it can't be seen; a closet, if possible, or even the bathroom. If you have a laundry room, why isn't it in there?

Now that you have a reading nook, take your books there. Stack them attractively next to your chaise or overstuffed chair to use as a table. They now have a purpose! If you find you've developed a collection (and that it's still growing), give the ones you can part with to a worthy cause, or a local second hand bookstore. Are you really going to read them again? Be honest!

Bedside table mess adds up quickly. That's especially true if your table doesn't have a place to tuck things away. The best bedside tables do. If yours doesn't, then maybe it's time for a change. Your medications don't really need to be within reach unless you suffer from a respiratory illness like asthma, or a heart condition. Tuck them away in a drawer, or better yet, put them in the medicine cabinet where they belong.

Take a critical look around your room. What else doesn't really need to be there? Is the ironing board set up, challenging you iron that pile of laundry? Fold it up and put it away. Is there a set of weights on the floor, gathering dust? Put them away. Whatever you can see that you don't need when you're sleeping needs to be put away, out of sight.

Your sacred sleeping space should induce a sense of calm, as you prepare to lay down for the night. It should be an oasis of peaceful order, not a moonscape of life's busyness and disarray.

Sacred is Sexy

While you may not think of sanctity in quite that way, "sanctity" can have more than one meaning. In this instance, it refers to a dedicated space set aside for only two purposes –

your sleep and your sexuality. Where you sleep is your sanctuary. It's private and it's all yours (to be shared with the one you love).

Your peaceful enclave is where only these two activities are appropriate. Everything else you do can be done somewhere else. Did you know that sex could contribute to a good night's rest?

Tell me that isn't the best news you've read all day!

Dr. Saralyn Mark, of the Yale School of Medicine relates that sex is a great way to improve your sleep because it elevates the level of oxytocin in your system. The presence of this hormone works to suppress cortisol production, which increases your stress level. If you're a woman, there's even more good news – increased estrogen production! Estrogen is a natural trigger for REM (Rapid Eye Movement) sleep, which is the deepest, most satisfying level of sleep you can get and the one we all need most.

In your newly peaceful, orderly sanctuary, what better medicine could there be to induce a good night's sleep than a little lovin'?

At least you'll have fun with the "clinical trials"!

Scentsual Sleep

There are certain scents that invigorate us. Others relax us. So why wouldn't your sacred sleep space benefit from some relaxing aromas? (These might also be welcome additions to those times you're engaging in the second activity permitted in your sanctuary)!

While you're preparing yourself for sleep (see "Sleep Hygiene") below, light a few scented candles here and there. Make sure these are placed with safety in mind.

Choose fragrances like lavender. This traditional aromatherapeutic sleep aid is especially effective for use by women. If lavender isn't your thing, try sandalwood, or bergamot. Dr. Bryan Raudenbush of Wheeling Jesuit University suggests jasmine. His study found that diffusing the scent of jasmine in the place study participants slept, led to them experience deeper sleep.

Any of the scents mentioned can be purchased in the form of essential oils. Add a few drops of any one of these to water in a spray bottle and spray your bed while you're preparing to lie down for the night.

Keep Your Cool

As discussed earlier in this book (see "Exercise"), your body temperature has an impact on how well you sleep. This is also true of the environment you sleep in.

Before turning in, set your thermostat to no more than 65 degrees (about 18 centigrade). If you can, crack your window just a little to allow air circulation. This measure will ensure that you're not breathing stale air as you sleep, but it will also keep your head cool, which is key to a good night's sleep.

In the summer months, invest in a fan. Position this as close to where you sleep as possible, without providing a further impediment to a good night's sleep (noise, motion).

Layer your bedding and always use a top sheet. Turn down the bedspread before retiring as part of your pre-sleep ritual and wear either lightweight pajamas, or none at all.

Keeping your bedroom as dark as possible (both day and night) is another great way to keep it cool. This measure also serves the purpose of blocking unnecessary light from outside at night. Heavy drapes or blinds will help you do this.

One-Third of Your Life – Worth an Investment

There's nothing more inviting than a beautifully dressed bed. While many of us minimize the importance of sheets, pillows, pillowcases and other accouterments for our beds, these can be another factor in getting a quality night's sleep.

High thread count sheets are soft and smooth against the skin. Quality pillows support our heads and necks, as we sleep. Quality bedding can beckon you from the other room and put a welcome dent in your nocturnal wakefulness, with its cushy allure.

Making the place you sleep as luxurious and comfortable as possible is not only a good strategy for improved rest; it's a gift to yourself and a reward after a long day.

Chapter 6: Sleep Hygiene

No matter what kind of day you've had; regardless of the challenges you've struggled with, bed time should become a ritual that signals your brain and body that the time has come to leave it all outside the door of your sleep sanctuary.

While we're often tempted to throw ourselves on the bed with no preparation of our bodies, or the place we're about to lay them for our night's rest, these habits don't serve us. Not engaging in a regular sleep hygiene regimen could be part of the reason we're not sleeping well.

Sleep hygiene forms a barrier between the world we move around in during the day and sleep. It forms a kind of psychological barrier between busyness and rest, and that can prove to be a strong support for improved sleep.

Here are a few of the boxes you need to check off to practice sound sleep hygiene:

- **Go to bed at the same time each night.** Get up at the same time each day. Establishing a sleeping pattern is a cornerstone of getting quality sleep.

- **Avoid stimulants in the evening.** Smoking cigarettes, as well as drinking alcohol and caffeine are habits to avoid in the hours before your appointed bedtime. The alcohol prohibition may seem counter-intuitive, but as your body assimilates alcohol, your sleep may be disrupted, later in the night.

- **Avoid eating after 8 pm.** This practice will also help you maintain you weight, or lose some you may have been wanting to.

Ritual is Restful

At an appointed hour each night, time should be set aside to physically prepare yourself for bed. By performing these self-care rituals each night, you are honoring your sleep time and giving it the prominence in your life it deserves.

Slow Down

Resist the temptation to engage in petty squabbles with loved ones or friends. Let your phone take a message. Don't check your email. It can all wait until tomorrow. Now might be the right time to take a few moments to write in your journal, or do the breathing exercises you've made a part of your daily life.

Your Very Own Turndown Service

Turn down your bed as you might expect it to be, were you staying in a fine hotel. Light a candle or two. If you've taken to spraying a relaxing scent on your bedclothes, do it now. Arrange your pillows the way you like them to be when you climb into bed.

Dress for Sleep Success

Remove your daytime clothing and put it away (as discussed earlier). If it needs to be washed, make sure it goes in the laundry basket. Change into clean sleeping attire in which you're comfortable and which is dedicated for wear *only* while you're sleeping.

Did You Brush Your Teeth?

I certainly hope so! I hope you also washed your face and brushed or combed your hair. Perhaps a soak in the tub, or a relaxing shower (depending on what works for you). Feeling that you've washed the day off has a finality to it that is another signal it's time to sleep.

It doesn't matter what order you perform these simple rituals in. Performing them as a prelude to sleeping is an effective way of letting your brain know that it's time. Setting aside the time to care for yourself before sleep will help you get the rest you need.

The Big "S"

Who admits to snoring? Almost everyone I know claims they don't snore. I used to, too. Then I woke myself up in mid-snore and all bets were off.

Snoring is a very common problem (so most of us are lying). It has broken up marriages and friendships, kept soldiers awake in barracks and students, in dormitories. It's estimated that almost half the population of the world snores. Of that percentage, 25% are regular sawers of logs. And this tendency is not, by any means, restricted to men! 20% of women snore, too!

But there is so much help now for this unfortunate condition that denial is only cheating those of us who snore out of a decent night's sleep.

Here are a few things you can do to reduce the likelihood of sawing logs that most of us would prefer not to hear sawed in the middle of the night:

- Don't sleep on your back. This sleeping position promotes snoring.

- Try not to smoke cigarettes (or at least, cut down).

- Reduce your alcohol intake.

- Try to lose a little weight (if you need to).

If you're already trying, or have tried employing these strategies and find they aren't helping, visit your General Practitioner to find out what else you might be doing.

There are so many ways to address this noisy (and annoying) problem and new therapies for snoring are being developed every day. In extreme cases, surgery may even be indicated. While that may sound drastic, eliminating this problem will pay off in sound sleep for you and those around you.

Check out the Resources section at the end of this book for

some useful information on therapies and devices that can put an end to or reduce habitual snoring.

Chapter 7: The Sleep Diet

As said before, the foods that you take in have a bigger impact on your sleeping patterns. Unhealthy diet i.e. the one comprised of processed foods and high-carb food may affect your hormonal balance and hinder effective sleep. These foods trigger production of ghrelin, a hormone that tells you to eat more and less of leptin that prevents over eating. Eating healthy foods can help relax the nervous system and restore sleep-inducing leptin in order for you fall asleep. Avoid eating foods high in sodium and sugar before bedtime as they cause dehydration, and replace them with vitamins and minerals-rich foods.

The rule of the thumb is to eat for your hormones. Ensure that you also eat within 30 minutes of waking up, though you don't have to eat a big breakfast. Consider a few eggs on whole-wheat toast or other food with high quality protein and complex carbs. If your schedule doesn't allow for cooking, then go for breakfast smoothie instead. If not sure of the foods to eat, these food groups should get you started on the path restful sleep.

1. Complex carbohydrates

Reach for foods such as brown rice, crackers, whole grain bread, pasta, and cereals. That said; avoid simple carbohydrates such as pastries, cookies, candies, white bread, sweet and other sugary foods. Processed foods can lower your serotonin levels and thus inhibit effective sleep. Try to eat whole grains as these contain an active ingredient referred to as tryptophan, very useful in brain relaxing serotonin. Whole grains also have magnesium, which researchers say can trigger stress and insomnia if lacking in the cells.

2. Lean proteins

You have various options such as fish, turkey, chicken and low fat cheese. Lean protein foods contain tryptophan, an amino acid that can raise your serotonin levels. On the contrary, avoid those deep-fried fish, high fat cheese, or chicken wings.

These foods take a long time to digest and hinder sleep since the metabolic activity is kept busy throughout. There are various sources for protein, which include:

- Fish: This includes catfish, salmon, trout, tuna, mackerel, and cod among other types of fish.

- White and red meat

  Birds are a great source of white meat, which supplies essential proteins. You can consume chicken, ducks, quails, turkey, or geese. Likewise, you can take pork as a source of white meat. For red meat, you can get it from goats, lamb, and cattle.

Other sources can include shellfish like oysters, lobsters, and crabs. Whole eggs, bacon, and sausages also act as very good sources of proteins. Protein powder can help supplement the amount of amino acids you get from meals. To use it, add it to your oatmeal or just bake it into recipes to ensure that you don't take excess carbs.

3. Heart-Healthy Fats

High fat diet isn't recommended though unsaturated fats are good at boosting serotonin levels and boost heart heath. Healthy fats include foods such as cashews, walnuts, pistachios, and pure peanut butter. Avoid those foods with saturated fats and Trans fats among them potato, French fries or other high-fat fries as they reduce your sleep-enhancing serotonin hormone.

Foods rich in these fats are rich in essential omega 3 fatty acids that help improve sleep and emotional wellbeing. A recent study confirmed that taking about 2.5 milligrams of omega-3 fatty acids for a period of 12 weeks could offer many benefits among them restful sleep. Cold-water and oily fishes like salmon are the most recommendable form of omega 3 you should look for. A 6-ounce piece of a grilled wild salmon has about 3.75 grams of omega 3. Other sources of amino acids include mussels, sardines, and anchovies.

4. Beverages

A few drinks such as a warm milk or peppermint tea drink can help promote sleep. If you need to drink caffeinated drinks, don't take coffee later than 2 PM to avoid having to wake up a few hours after drinking. Another option is to drink a fresh cup of green tea, which has effective properties and actually works by crossing against your brain barriers. Green tea also contains an active substance known as L-theanine. This ingredient has been studied and found to boost mood, improve sleep and calm nerves, and doesn't cause any side effects.

When you drink green tea, it boosts serotonin enhancing transmitters among them dopamine. To make a healthy drink of green tea, just boil a cup of water and add a green tea bag. Combine the two and drink preferably in the morning as part of your breakfast.

5. Fresh Herbs And Spices

Research has shown that various herbs can help calm your body among them basil and sage due to their tension reducing chemicals found in them. You can easily prepare a homemade pasta sauce using basil and sage, as this version has low sugar content compared to commercial sauces. On the contrary, do not include black or red pepper since they have a stimulatory impact on your sleep. Also try out these herbs:

- Chamomile

This tea contains flavonoids, an active substance that allows chamomile to relax a troubled mind and fall asleep. The herb helps relax your muscles, due to the presence of a chemical called apigenin, which has the ability to bid GABA receptors and cause sleepiness. You can either buy chamomile from local stores or prepare your own fresh variety.

Actually, you only need 2 teaspoons of dried chamomile and a cup of boiling water. Boil your water and then add dried chamomile. Allow the tea steep for about 5 minutes or additional 10 minutes if using a tea bag. Strain the tea, add some honey or milk if desired, and drink 30 minutes to bed. In case you're using the fresh flowers, just choose the heads and compost the stems.

- Valerian

Lack of sleep can be effectively treated with naturally occurring valerian herb that functions better than traditional sleeping pills and eliminates side effects. Valerian herb contains isovaltrate, an active ingredient responsible for its medicinal properties. The herb works by boosting the amount of gamma aminobutryic acid, which is known to control the action of nerve cells and to calm nerves. Using the herb will relive you from problems such as insomnia, sleeplessness, and restless nights, as valerian root has a sedative and soothing impact.

Valerian root is recommendable, as it does not cause sleepiness or drowsiness during daytime. The root also acts as a muscle relaxant and can be used to effectively reduce muscle cramps and spasms. You can easily brew your own valerian tea from these ingredients:

-8 oz. fresh water, hot from the tap

-8 oz. fresh water to boil

-Strainer or infusion device, say a tea ball

-1 teaspoon of dried valerian root

Fill a cup or mug to steep tea in the hot water. Boil about 8 ounce of water in a kettle bottle, remove it from the heat and then empty the mug that contains hot water. Put a teaspoon of valerian root into the mug and pour in the hot water. Cover the mixture and allow to steep for around 15 minutes, then uncover and strain. To add flavor, include a little honey or milk and then sip few hours before bed.

- Lemon balm

Lemon has traditionally been used as a cure for stress and anxiety for many years, and it can also help with insomnia. The lemon scented herb is a plant from the mint family and has been proven to boost sleep especially when coupled with herbs like valerian. Based on a study, more than 8 percent of participants who took lemon balm and valerian herbal drink experienced many improvements in sleeping patterns. Though you can buy both as dietary supplements, try making your own drink from a teaspoon root of valerian and 1-2 teaspoons of dried lemon balm. Add the mixture to a cup of hot water and steep for around 5-10 minutes. However, ensure you talk to a doctor in case you are under other medication to prevent possible counter reaction.

Also obtain:

-8 ounces of fresh water

-2 teaspoons dried chamomile

-Some honey

--10 tablespoons fresh or 2 tablespoons of dried lemon balm

Put the loose herbs into a mug and then add 8 ounces boiling water. Then steep for around 5 minutes, strain and enjoy the drink around 30-45 minutes before retiring to bed.

If you can't get the actual herb, lemon balm is also sold as a tincture, capsule and tea. You can use it in combination with other calming herbs like valerian, chamomile, and hops. While lemon balm is considered safe to take, it has been shown that taking too much of it can actually increase your anxiety. The best approach is to start slowly and follow the recommended dosage.

- **Saint John's Wort**

The herb contains hypercine, an active ingredient that helps boost the level of serotonin in the brain. The higher the level of serotonin, the more the melatonin produced and the better the quality of sleep. The herb can be consumed in capsule form, but you can also prepare your own from fresh ingredients:

-Honey or lemon

-8 ounces boiled water

-2 teaspoons of dried herb

To prepare, put the Saint John's Wort herb into a mug and then cover it with freshly boiled water. Steep the tea for about 5 minutes, strain and then drink around an ounce daily. Try taking 30-45 minutes before bedtime.

- Lavender

The herb is useful as a sleep aid both as brewed tea and as an essential oil that can be distilled from its leaves, the stem, and flowers of the plant. You can either apply lavender topically to relax tense muscles or instead inhale the calming aroma for similar calming benefit. For instance, you can rub the essential oil topically on the feet as a way to get easily absorbed into the body. To inhale, simply add to your bath water, a vaporizer or bad it into a tissue and breathe into it. In other cases, try making a sachet from its flowers and leaves and place it underneath the bed before you sleep.

However, when applying the lavender externally, be aware of allergic reaction thus you should do a patch test before application. Get a teaspoon of fresh or ½ teaspoon of dried lavender alongside 2 teaspoons of dried mint. You can also incorporate other herbs like rose geranium, lemon verbena, lemon balm, or rosemary. To prepare, mix together mint and lavender into a saucepan and then pour a cup of boiling water over the mixture. Then steep for 5 minutes and strain to enjoy.

To make homemade lavender sachet gather the following:

- Ribbon (1/4" wide)

- Thread

-1 regular size needles

-1 large needle to fit 1/4" ribbon

-A handkerchief

-Lavender essential oil

-Lavender plant (stems, leaves or buds)

Start by folding the handkerchief into half, and then fold it into half again. Then sew 3 sides into half using a sewing machine or just a needle and thread. Open the unsown side of your handkerchief and fill it with the lavender buds or other plant parts. You should use a lot of plant material but ensure that it's not too tight, in order to look like a beanbag.

Sprinkle the plant pieces with 8-10 drops of lavender essential oil and then thread the large needle with ¼ inch ribbon. Ensure you loosely thread in order to keep the plant materials inside the DIY sachet. Tie the whole sachet with a knot and then place it underneath your bed before sleeping.

- Hops

This vine has the potential to calm your nerves and make you relax into sleep. You can make a strong tea of hops herb or place a sleep sachet under your pillow at night. Gather the following 4 cups of boiling water and 2 tablespoons of dried hops. Place the hops into a quart glass jar and then cover using boiling water. Let it steep while tightly covered for 5 hours or overnight, before you strain. To use, you can reheat and drink one cup 30-45 minutes before bed. Refrigerate the rest for about 2 days.

- Catnip

This plant comes from the mint family and has shown to offer relaxing properties due to the presence of nepetalactone compound. The herb can facilitate relaxation and cause drowsiness when taken before bed. You should make a cup of warm herbal tea with a little honey to taste. Add 4 teaspoons of fresh or 1-2 teaspoons of dried catnip into 8 ounces of boiling water. Steep the mixture for 10 minutes, uncover and then add in some honey. Drink the tea around 30 minutes before bed.

- Ginseng

The herb is useful in improving sleep, boosting your mental performance and improving memory. Ginseng is also effective in treating mental symptoms like anxiety, stress, and depression. The herb consists of an active ingredient referred to as ginsenosides, which enables the herb to cure stress and fight lack of sleep. If seeking to look younger and active, the herb helps lower blood degeneration.

- Passionflower

This is a sedative herb and has been approved for nervous restlessness and stress-related problems like insomnia. Like any other sedative, passionflower can cause drowsiness and sleepiness when taken alongside a prescription sedative. Take caution when using multiple herbs or home remedies at the same time.

- Kava root

The herb has been proven to treat a number of conditions among them stress, anxiety and insomnia. The herb can also help to relax your mind and offer you the peaceful rest that has proven hard to achieve.

- Wild lettuce

You can obtain this herb, which can treat insomnia and restlessness. The herb is available in a couple of formulas meant to treat chronic and acute insomnia. It's very safe and calming for both adults and children. You'll need a daily dosage of 2-3 drops of herbal tincture, about 3-4 times daily.

- California poppy

This sedative is known to promote sleep and help you relax. The herb is a mild analgesic and can thus be administered to children without causing complications. The herb has been studied for potencies against anxiety and sleeplessness. You'll require about a cup of California poppy about 1-3 times daily, or 30-40 drops of a tincture daily.

- Chaste tree

This herb has shown to treat insomnia or other sleep-related conditions. Women who suffer from severe premenstrual syndrome are more likely to get relief from this herb. The herb can treat PMS-related insomnia that also features other conditions like abdominal cramping.

6. Healthy Snacks

Be sure to have healthy snacks in your meal plan. Healthy snacks contain important minerals and vitamins that can increase the level of hormones that will enhance your sleep. Eating unhealthy snacks prevents you from taking what you actually need to fall asleep, and can even result in unpleasant side effects such as headaches that can leave you in a bad mood. Before bed or taking a nap, you can eat snacks such as whole grain crackers, an apple, some brown rice, almond batter or low-fat mozzarella string cheese. Other sleep-promoting snacks include 100-percent whole grain crackers smeared with peanut butter, low fat yoghurt and banana as well as low-fat cottage cheese topped with whole grain pita chips.

Foods That Boost Sleep

Foods that work to boost the quality of sleep are rich in a substance called tryptophan. This nutrient is known to boost the levels of serotonin, which is a precursor to melatonin, a hormone that triggers sleep. Melatonin is described as that hormone that controls your circadian rhythm and controls your natural sleep cycles. Both melatonin and tryptophan can help activate various brain chemicals and this helps to encourage restful sleep.

That said, you should eat these foods, as they are rich in sleep inducing tryptophan and others nutrients that your body requires to functions optimally:

- Dark chocolate

The pure dark variety of chocolate can boost mood, sleep, as well as relieve stress. This is because it reduces cortisol, a stress hormone that leads to anxiety-like symptoms; i.e. sleeplessness. The stress hormone can also lead to other problems like weight gain and fatigue; and can prevent relaxation. However, only reach for the pure variety that has no added sugars. Also reduce the amount of dark chocolate you consume since it has a little amount of caffeine which can interfere with sleep.

- Almonds

These nuts are rich in both calcium and magnesium, and can be a good snack option. Almonds contain zinc, which can help to control or balance your mood. They also possess iron and healthy fats. Iron is important since it helps prevent brain fatigue that leads to both anxiety and a lack of energy.

Almonds are also known to provide protein that can maintain your blood sugar level as you sleep, alongside switching the body from the alert adrenaline cycle into the rest-and-digest cycle. You may decide to either eat a handful of these nutritious nuts or instead spread your whole grain bread with some almond butter! Try eating 1-ounce portion of almonds or a teaspoon of almond butter as your bedtime snack.

- Pumpkin seeds

These seeds contain healthy fats, needed to improve sleep and boost your mood. Pumpkin seeds contains L-tryptophan, which is an amino acid required to produce serotonin neurotransmitters. To get this benefit, obtain a cup of pumpkin seeds per day, and sprinkle it with some salt.

- Blueberries

They might not be your preferred fruits but are rich in vitamins and plant nutrients known as phytonutrients. They also contain antioxidants, substances, which help relieve stress and anxiety.

- Cherries

Cherries exist in various varieties and research has confirmed that all do have a high quality melatonin hormone that helps induce sleep. In a scientific study, people who drank about 8 ounces of tart cherry juice both in the morning and in the evening witnessed improved sleep quality within 2 weeks. To realize these benefits, try to consume a cup of whole cherries as your late night snack, which works in a similar manner as cherry juice.

- Fish

This protein-rich food has high amount of tryptophan, a natural sedative; with fish like tuna, cod, and shrimp having the highest amounts compared to turkey. Fish such as salmon, halibut, and tuna are also rich in vitamin B6 which is required by the body to manufacture serotonin and melatonin. Also try crustaceans like Shrimp and Lobster as these are rich in tryptophan too. However, to ensure that you eat only clean seafood, only stick to those fish like Pole-caught tuna from US or the Pacific cod from Alaska. Other foods with vitamin B6 include pistachio nuts and raw garlic.

- Bananas

These fruits can work well as snack foods, and are recommended due to the high amounts of magnesium and potassium. These two minerals are known to improve mood and promote relaxation. Various research studies have shown that magnesium deficiencies can cause nighttime muscle cramps and restless leg syndrome, conditions that inhibit sleep. To realize the efficiency of the fruit, ensure that you eat at least a banana daily. You can also prepare bedtime smoothie by blending a cup of milk or soymilk with one banana.

- Spinach

The veggie is praised due to high magnesium and potassium content but is still rich in calcium, a mineral that controls sleep. Calcium works by facilitating the body to produce melatonin, in a bid to restore the optimum circadian rhythm. Spinach also has a particular nutrient called glutamine, which is considered as a precursor in neurotransmitter pathways that can help monitor sleep-wake cycles. If you don't like eating spinach, you can get similar benefits from veggies like turnip greens, kale, Swiss chard, collard greens and other leafy green veggies.

- Miso Soup

Next time you visit your restaurant, order an 8-ounce of this nutritious broth to help improve your sleep quality. Miso has amino acids, which can boost the synthesis of melatonin, and can fight other infections that affect better sleep such as occasional cold.

- Dairy

Dairy products do have calcium that boosts melatonin level, with products like cheese; milk and yoghurt having been proven to contain tryptophan. Calcium can help reduce stress levels and stabilize your nerve fibers, especially those located in the brain. Research studies have concluded that calcium deficiency can lead to poor sleep.

The calcium in foods like cheese and crackers can help the brain to utilize tryptophan to make sleep-inducing tryptophan. The mineral also helps regulate your muscle movements. Yogurt can help boost the level of good bacteria or probiotics in your gut, and boost the quality o sleep. To improve the quality of sleep, try drinking a cup of Greek yoghurt before bed. Alternatively, you can drink about a glass of warm milk a few hours before sleep to boost melatonin levels.

- Oatmeal

Known as a good breakfast option, oatmeal can help enhance rest and improve sleep. The oats are rich in potassium, phosphorus, magnesium, and calcium; all minerals that help suppress stress and boost sleep. However, don't try to add any sweeteners to the oatmeal especially before bedtime as this can affect the calming ability in oatmeal. If you really like your sweet tooth try to top with sleep inducing fruits like bananas.

- Edamame

Especially for women who often crave for a bedtime snack, try a lightly salted edamame; as it contains estrogen-like substances that help control nighttime hot flashes that interferes with sleep. You can opt for a recipe like blending 2 cups of shelled and cooked edamame, with a clove of garlic, a drizzle of olive oil and teaspoon of salt.

- Hard-Cooked Egg

High in proteins, eggs can help boost the amount of tryptophan in your blood plasma. To enjoy the benefits that come from eggs, try baking an egg and then combine it with leftovers or other foods for breakfast. Also try a mushroom and spinach frittata and ensure that you include egg yolks as they are rich in tyrosine and tryptophan which offer antioxidant properties. You need antioxidants to kill free radicals that damage cells and interfere with metabolic activities.

- Pineapples

The fruit has a good amount of bromelain, a type of protein that can help fight night coughs and ensure you relax for a good night's sleep. Try mixing together coconut and pineapple to prepare recipes with chicken or other ingredients.

- Tofu

Most soy products are known to contain tryptophan that helps boost the quality of sleep. The good thing is that you can substitute any protein food with tofu and incorporate in many vegan or vegetarian recipes. For instance, try making a tofu kebab that features bell peppers and ginger for additional nutrients.

- Turkey

This meat has tryptophan, which is well known to boost sleep. Try making various turkey recipes say Asian turkey rice bowl or other favorite meals.

- Walnuts

The nuts are also rich in tryptophan, an amino acid that helps to boost melatonin and serotonin levels in the brain. Actually, walnuts have their own source of melatonin, and thus are preferred to induce sleep within a few minutes of consuming.

- Lettuce

The veggie contains lactucarium, a sedative that can help soothe the brain in a similar manner as opium. Try to simmer 3-4 large lettuce leaves in a cup of water for around 15 minutes. Turn the heat off and then top with a sprig of mint, and then sip before you retire to bed. Alternatively, a salad of lettuce and other green veggies should also do the trick.

- Pretzels

It's a fact that foods like corn chips and pretzels have a high glycemic index and can therefore spike your blood glucose and insulin levels. Majority of experts recommend that you should have a steady level of blood glucose and insulin to avoid effects such as insulin resistance and mood swings. However, if interested in boosting sleep, be aware that increase in insulin and blood glucose levels can help raise tryptophan levels in the blood. You may not believe it but this can shorten the time it takes for you to fall asleep!

- Rice

Research has shown that low levels of glucose can interfere with sleep, thus you need to consume a carbohydrate meal and high protein meal before going to bed. Both carbs and proteins can help raise the level of glucose in the blood and make you fall asleep faster. Try to mix the two food groups to increase amount of insulin released, to facilitate tryptophan to break through brain barriers.

Aim for high glycemic index foods like white rice, as it can help reduce the time you take to fall asleep. For instance, a recent study confirmed that eating jasmine rice could help improve sleep. Participants who took the rice before retiring to bed were found to sleep faster than those who consumed other rice types.

- Passion-fruit Tea

A study by Australian researchers found out that taking a cup of passion fruit at least 1 hour before bed could help boost quality of sleep. The fruit contains a substance called Harman alkaloids, which work on the brain to make it tired and restful.

- Honey

Honey contains a natural sugar, which can increase the level of insulin, to facilitate the insulin in blood to enter the brain. Try taking a spoon of honey or combine it with chamomile tea for better action.

- Kale

Majority of leafy dark green veggies such as kales are rich in calcium, a mineral that helps the brain to utilize tryptophan to produce sleep-inducing melatonin. If you don't like kales, try mustard greens or spinach for calcium and other nutrients.

- Hummus

These chickpeas contain high amount of tryptophan. Chickpeas also contain vitamin B6, which has ability to synthesize its own melatonin. Eating a light lunch of hummus alongside grain crackers can actually help you obtain that afternoon nap or night sleep you want.

- Elk

This game meat has been proven to contain twice the amount of tryptophan compared to turkey breast. Try eating this meat with a side dish of carb rich foods to help the tryptophan from meat to reach the brain.

- Juice

Since you are restricted from drinking drinks like coffee and other caffeine containing beverages, why not drink juice instead? Just swap that afternoon coffee with juice enriched with fresh herbs and spices to boost the level of anti-oxidants in the blood. Before retiring to bed, try to blend a cup of basil, a cup of parsley, 3 cups of broccoli, 5 cups kales, 4 cups lettuce, 5 cups spinach and about 8 tablespoons of fresh lemon juice.

- Broccoli

The veggie is rich in various vitamins like vitamin A, C and K that help the body to function optimally. Research has shown that lack of these minerals can interfere with normal routine like restful sleep. Broccoli also has high quality fiber, iron, protein, and magnesium, which have shown to boost sleep.

- Bell Peppers

The peppers have vitamin C, which helps boost sleep, alongside fighting infections that inhibit effective sleep. Peppers can provide the energy you need to remain active and prevent you from feeling weary at night. Ensure that you add in some bell peppers into your lunch salad or afternoon snack for better outcome.

- Strawberries

These berries contain vitamins and anti-oxidants and are less acidic compared to similar fruits like oranges. The acidity in citrus fruits can cause acid reflux or heart burn and thus cannot be advisable for night-time snack. Strawberries are healthy when made into a smoothie, juice, or added to other snacks and don't cause problems such as weight gain.

- Watermelon

The fruit is rich in lycopene, a nutrient that gives it the healthy and sleep-inducing properties. Watermelon is a super-food, and is available all year round.

- Dates

These contain both carbs and tryptophan and thus they promote drowsiness and are able to work more effectively. Research has shown that eating dates 1 hour before bed can help you reduce the time you spend falling asleep. Eat dates for both benefits.

- Grapefruit

The fruit has lycopene, an antioxidant that promotes sleep. Furthermore, the fruit can also help you shed pounds and prevent heart disease.

- Tomatoes

Known for their high amount of lycopene, tomatoes are a good option for salads, smoothies and other meals. However, cooked tomatoes have higher level of lycopene thus try to cook them to boost the anti-oxidant levels. Add a few tomatoes to your dishes to boost sleep; fight cancer and improve your general life.

- Saffron

Look for that orange red saffron which has the best flavor and mood enhancing effect. A recent study found out that water-based extract of saffron could help boost sleep time and reduce weight gain.

Dietary Tips To Fight Sleeplessness

One of the best tips to enhance sleep is to eat calcium and magnesium rich foods or supplements to help relax your muscles. This can go a long way into making you fall asleep. Some great sources of calcium and magnesium are green leafy veggies or a drink of warm milk during dinner. In addition, indulge in a protein rich and carbohydrate rich diet with plenty of amino acid to help relax and calm your mind and body. On the other hand, avoid eating rich and heavy foods at least 2 hours before you sleep since fatty food take a lot of time before your stomach can digest it, which may keep you awake.

Try the following dietary advice:

- Eat a healthy breakfast

Eating a healthy and balanced diet is important to refresh your bodily functions and encourage healthy sleeping patterns later in the night. It is important to start the day with a healthy breakfast to get you going. Research has shown that the kind of food you take in the morning can have a tremendous effect on your sleep patterns. If you are not careful, eating certain foods can aggravate your sleeplessness and other stress-related symptoms. This includes beverages such as coffee, tea, soft drinks, soda, and fast foods.

Eating a healthy breakfast in the morning makes you feel rejuvenated and are able to tackle the day's challenges actively. You are able to deal with some of life's stresses, fight lack of sleep at night, and develop a healthier mind too. That said; ensure that you incorporate the right foods in your diet. Breakfast in particular should be heavy and lunch a little light. A healthy breakfast will re-energize you and help you concentrate throughout the day. When choosing your breakfast, you need to be aware of these things:

1. Magnesium should be present in your diet to avoid cases of chronic fatigue, insomnia, and restless leg syndrome. High magnesium content foods include green vegetables and seeds such as sunflower and pumpkin.

2. Incorporate enough proportion of proteins. These foods contain amino acid tryptophan, which influences the level of serotonin, a chemical substance that controls mood, sleep, and cognitive function.

3. Lack of iron in the body can lead to excessive fatigue, which can cause sleeplessness. Foods rich in iron include eggs, whole grains, and vegetables.

4. Vitamin B12 is vital for various chemical processes such as DNA synthesis and the production of the red blood cells. Having a deficiency of it can cause lack of sleep and accelerated stress levels.

5. If you fail to have enough vitamin D in your body, you will experience symptoms of insomnia, fatigue, and muscle pain. Taking foods rich in vitamin D for your breakfast such as fortified milk, liver and calcium supplements can boost your vitamin D levels tremendously.

- Eliminate sugar

Be aware that incorporating too much sugar can contribute to hormonal imbalances which can affect your sleep. You also need to reduce the amounts of fruits that you consume. Though it's advisable to eat a number of servings of fruits daily, majority of fruits are rich in fructose that is unhealthy for the body. For instance, modern apples, which had 2 grams of fructose have been hybridized for sweetness, yielding apples with 20-25 grams of fructose. Ensure that you keep away from high fructose and instead focus on natural fats such as avocados and olives for hormone reset.

Eat lean proteins, healthy and unsaturated fatty acids and high fiber foods such as legumes, low-glycemic fruits and leafy greens. Eating whole foods can help you optimize your hormonal levels as well as burn more fats. In numerous scientific studies, obese and overweight women were found to lose more fat with whole foods and with boosted hormonal levels.

- Consume more amino acids

As opposed to taking supplements, dietary protein has proved to stabilize insulin and optimize related hormones. You can get 35 percent of muscle protein by obtaining branched chain amino acids such as valine, isoleucine and leucine. Taking these BCAAs before exercising can boost your sleep hormone and improve your general health. Obtain your high-quality amino acids from free-range poultry, wild-caught fish, and grass-fed beef. If you don't prefer protein from meat sources, go for high-quality plant based proteins from raw nuts, quinoa and legumes. Also try protein prodders especially those made from grass-fed whey or pea.

- Monitor poly-unsaturated fats

Vegetable oils have high amounts of poly-unsaturated fats, which the body doesn't need for hormone production or making new cells. When you consume excess omega 6 fatty acids, the body is forced to utilize the polyunsaturated fat for cell repair and generation. These fats are very unstable and can oxidize when exposed to light or into the body and thus cause mutation and inflammation in cells. This affects how your body functions and can interfere with normal activities like restful sleeping.

Avoid vegetable oils, shortening, margarine, soybean oil, canola oil, peanuts, and other chemical processed fats. The healthiest fat to go for is olive oil, real butter, coconut oil, and animal fats such as lard or tallow. Ensure that fats come from healthy sources and are rich in omega 3 fatty acids.

- Limit the Caffeine

Majority of people like coffee, but bear in mind that excess amounts of caffeine can affect the endocrine system. Caffeine is blamed for increasing cortisol hormone level and thus wrecks the nervous system. With high amounts of the hormone, your body is stressed and this has a great impact on your sleep patterns.

Reduce the amount of coffee as much as possible, and replace its consumption with herbal teas. If it's hard cutting down on black coffee for instance, try adding a tablespoon of coconut oil to each cup and then blend to emulsify. You'll get healthy fats and reduce effect of caffeine to your system. To control the production of cortisol hormone, try using holy basil herb that comes as a capsule. You can also eat cortisol-fighting foods such as barley, beans, nuts, citrus, and spinach.

- Take proper supplements to reset your hormones

Vitamins and other nutrients control how your body functions including your sleep patterns, metabolism and circulation process. Your body requires sufficient amounts of vitamin D and magnesium for optimal hormonal functioning. However, where these nutrients cannot be obtained from diet, you can consider supplements to bridge the gaps. Look for those supplements that support hormone reset such as:

Magnesium

The nutrient is important for hundreds of processes in your body and in helping you get good sleep. The most effective magnesium supplement is ionic liquid form that can be added to foods and drinks and then adjust the dose slowly with time. There's also trans-dermal magnesium that is directly applied to the skin and is a very effective remedy for women with severe magnesium deficiency or damaged digestive tract.

Maca

This tuber belongs to radish family, and is attributed to boosting hormone production especially for better sleep. The tuber also has high amounts of fatty acids and minerals, thus it's recommended for hormone reset. The supplement is available in capsule or much cheaper powder form.

Vitamin D

This a pre-hormone that supports optimum function of hormones, and can be best obtained from sunlight. As a supplement, it's available as D3.

Fermented Cod Liver Oil

It offers the required building blocks for hormones such as vitamin A, D and K. Cod liver oil is also a rich source of healthy fats like omega 3 fatty acids.

5-htp

This is a supplement that is also referred to as 5-hydroxytryptophan, meant to restore a natural tryptophan amino acid. The supplement comes from the seed extract of *Griffonia simplicifolia*. 5-htp is a serotoninprecursor and helps boost serotonin levels in the brain, needed for regulation of sleep. The 5-htp can easily penetrate the bloodstream into the brain and facilitate a natural calm that promote sleep.

- Monitor dairy products

Dairy products cause hormonal imbalances. Avoid dairy products from cattle injected with steroid hormones meant to fatten it. Milk, fat, or cheese from such animals is toxic and leads to disruption of hormones. It's recommended to reach for milk alternatives among them coconut milk, almond milk and coconut kefir.

Chapter 8: Other Natural Remedies That Boost Sleep

- Melatonin

You can get melatonin in supplements form meant to address sleeplessness. The body produces this naturally to help monitor the sleep-wake cycle of the brain when the light exposure reduces at night. Melatonin can also be administered in supplements especially if you suffer serious sleep disorders. The supplements can help raise sleep quality and improve morning alertness according to research. You need to take melatonin supplements at about 2 hours before sleep for a period of 8 weeks. Actually even lower doses of 0.1-0.3 mg melatonin hormone can function in a similar way as higher dose of 3-5mg. However, don't take in the morning as this can delay your circadian rhythm and slow down your productivity.

- Light Exposure

Exposure to light in the morning is an important thing if you have delayed sleep-phase syndrome or other sleep deficiency condition. Lights communicate to the body and trigger production of melatonin at night and instruct the body to wake up. Experts say that about 30 minutes walk outdoors first thing in the morning or an alternative light therapy can help improve sleep. For those who wake up too early, it's advisable to get exposed to light during the late afternoons. Try to have a walk outdoors for about 2-3 hours in the evening. You can look for light therapy units or have one suggested to you by your sleep specialist or a doctor.

- Acupuncture

This procedure is based on the belief that inserting needles at specific trigger points can help make patients relax and fall asleep. Acupuncture is known to activate your body's natural energy flow and restores internal balance. The technique is believed to correct imbalances in the flow of your energy called "qi" in channels referred to as meridians. The thin needles inserted into the body are believed to open the blocked channels and thus facilitate the brain to understand the moment you need to sleep. It does so by signaling the production of melatonin or tryptophan to facilitate fast and restful sleep. There are other methods of stimulating the acu-points on the body such as application of pressure, heat and laser light.

Chapter 9: Helpful Sleep Tips

The importance of sleep is already well known to you by now. However, the information you have received so far has been quite detailed and expansive, thus making it hard to figure out how to properly implement it in your daily routines. This chapter is dedicated to providing bite sized tips that you can apply in order to get the best sleep possible. These tips are uncomplicated and easy to follow, and should be able to provide an easy solution for you to improve the quality of your sleep and regulate your sleep patterns.

Avoid Stimulants and Depressants

We tend to consume a significant number of stimulants as well as depressants over the course of our daily routines. From coffee to wake us up in the morning to alcohol to help us unwind; there are a number of different substances we consume that alter the way our body is feeling. When you count activities such as smoking, you have a definite recipe for restless nights.

Coffee and cigarettes fill your body with chemicals that make you feel active. These chemicals are largely responsible for the buzz you feel after consuming these things. If you drink coffee, strong tea or smoke a cigarette about six hours before you sleep, you are going to end up spending the night awake because your body will be unable to shut down.

Based on research for instance, caffeine takes about 12 hours to be eliminated from the body. If you drink coffee during afternoon snack time, you'll at least knock off 1 hour of sleep time. There are people who drink coffee just because they didn't sleep well the previous night but instead fall into a vicious cycle. Coffee will 'rob' your sleep, make you tired, and reduce your productivity. Likewise, alcohol can affect your sleep patterns especially after its sedative properties wears off.

Alcohol doesn't help either. Consuming alcohol makes you sleepy, but you don't get as much REM sleep if your body is filled with alcohol. As a result, you are not going to have restful sleep and are going to be tired the next day.

Your Bedroom Should be for Sleep

These days, our bedrooms have become hubs of activity. With so much technology at our disposal using which we can stay connected to the world around us even in the comfort of our own bedrooms, it has become very common for us to do a number of things in our sleeping rooms apart from getting shuteye.

This makes your brain associate your room with a lot of different things apart from sleep. As a result, if you go to sleep and are not absolutely flat out exhausted you are going to start thinking about the different things you can do while you are in your bedroom. You are going to want to check your phone, watch some TV, read a book, and all of these things are going to interfere with your ability to maintain a regular sleep cycle.

Therefore, keep the bedroom for sleep and sex. If you must perform other activities in bed or in your bedroom, try to make them calm activities. Don't watch loud sports games while in bed, or action packed movies. Try reading a relaxing book instead, something that is going to end up facilitating sleep.

Create an Ideal Sleeping Environment

Everybody has their own preferences when it comes to an ideal sleeping environment. If you tend to feel the heat more than most people, you might like your room to be cold while you are trying to sleep. If you prefer to sleep without a blanket whenever possible you might want to avoid turning your air conditioner on while sleeping.

Some people need pitch darkness in order to be able to sleep properly. Other people prefer some form of soft light, especially if they are afraid of the dark. There are others still who simply don't care; sleep comes to them regardless of the amount of light in their surroundings.

What all of this means is that you need to discover what your sleeping preferences are. You probably know what makes you comfortable enough to sleep, but on the off chance that you don't, try experimenting. Try soft light instead of pitch darkness; try turning the air conditioner or heater off. Some people just can't sleep if their room is being artificially cooled or heated as it changes the texture of the air. Once you have discovered your ideal sleeping environment, try to make your room consistently meet these requirements.

For instance, you can also incorporate aromatherapy into your bedroom through cedar-wood and lavender essential oil as these trigger your sleep senses. Add a few drops of water to constitute linen spray for the pillows, or rub on the soles of the feet. Another option is to lower temperature down or turn the clock away from your view, as watching your sleep time has shown to cause anxiety and delayed sleep. In case you reside in a noisy environment, you can consider making the house sound proof or alternatively play soothing sounds from apps to help drain that noise.

Follow a Pre-Sleep Routine

Human beings are creatures of habit. We tend to get bored if habit becomes the norm, but as far as things that are as natural as sleep are concerned, regularity is a very positive sign.

One reason that you might not be able to sleep properly is if your mind is unable to ascertain when it is supposed to start shutting down. With more and more of us taking work home and working well in the wee hours of the night, it has become common for people to go to sleep right after finishing work.

This results in the brain being unable to switch itself off for a while because it had been in overdrive for so long. It gets confused at the sudden shift in environment and thus takes a while to lull you off to sleep.

This is why it is important to have a pre-sleep routine. This will help your brain realize that it is time for sleep so that it can start slowing down the amount of work that it is doing and preparing for shut down. Think of your brain as a computer. Simply unplugging it can damage it; you need to shut it down properly.

A pre-sleep routine can include a number of different activities. One of the most popular is meditation. Try meditating for a few minutes, say about ten to fifteen, after you are done with work and are about to go to sleep. Another popular pre-bedtime activity is reading. Both of these activities require low brain activity while keeping it stimulated, thus allowing it to power down slowly.

By turning these activities into a habit, you will eventually be able to use them as a signal of sorts to tell your brain that it is time to power down and go to sleep.

Avoid Looking at the Clock

It is understandable. You have work in the morning, and are stressed out about the fact that you are unable to sleep. As a result, you keep looking at the clock, wanting to know just how much time you have left before you have to get up in the morning.

However, just because something is understandable does not mean that it is healthy. By constantly looking at the clock, you are going to be doing two things.

✓ Firstly, you are going to be keeping your brain active by looking at the light of the clock. Forcing it to focus removes any chance it has to shut down. It's like when your computer screen is going black but you move your mouse. It will only light back up again, and the whole shut down cycle will begin anew.

✓ Secondly, the stress of wondering what the time is could keep you up. Your brain will remain active, trying to process the stress you are feeling, constantly thinking about how long you have left to sleep.

Hence, it would be helpful to just avoid looking at the clock altogether. A good idea would be to remove clocks from your bedroom altogether.

Avoid Screens before Bedtime

The blessing and curse of the modern man is that we have become so connected to one another. The presence of smart phones makes our lives a lot easier, but at the same time owning a smart phone might end up getting you addicted to looking at the screen, trying to see if you have any new notifications or messages.

This is a natural part of every person's routine, but it is not healthy to do right before you sleep. At that time, your mind requires peace. The reason most of us prefer sleeping when it's dark is that it helps our brains recognize that it is night, the time of day when the vast majority of us are programmed to sleep.

By looking at your smart phone screen or any other similar device, you are going to end up tricking your brain into thinking that it is still daytime. This would result in your brain taking far longer to get to sleep, as well as making it less likely that you will be able to achieve REM sleep.

Maintain a Consistent Schedule

This is yet another curse brought about by modern conveniences. We have so much artificial light in our lives that our internal clocks have become all but useless. This is why it has become more important than ever to maintain a proper schedule, one that you follow regardless of whether it is a weekend or a weekday.

This means going to bed at the same time and waking up at the same time every day. By going to bed at the same time every night, you are going to program your body into recognizing a time of day when it is supposed to start shutting down and preparing for sleep. Having an inconsistent sleep time would result in you being unable to sleep until your eyes are actually falling shut against your will.

Try to maintain a morning routine as well. This will act as a signal to tell your body that it is time to awaken and properly initiate all of its various functions. The benefit of this is that it will further allow you to create demarcation between the time of day when you are supposed to sleep and when you are supposed to wake up.

Take a Nap

Some people tend to believe that taking naps is bad for your sleep cycle. This is based on fairly sound logic. After all, by napping you are fulfilling part of your body's sleep quota. Ostensibly, this would mean that when you lie down to sleep at night your body would be too fresh from your nap to be able to shut down quickly.

Naps are actually wonderful for your sleep cycle. They give you energy in the middle of the day, allowing your body to take a bit of a breather. They also help regulate the chemicals in your brain, facilitating a more relaxed mind when you finally lay down to sleep.

However, keep in mind that the timing of your naps is very important. Taking naps later on during the day might ruin your sleep cycle because in this case your body *will* be associating the nap with your regular sleep time and chalking the amount of time you nap off of your sleep quota in disproportionate amounts.

Hence, if you are napping try to do so not too long after midday, and make sure that your nap lasts no longer than thirty minutes.

Keep Hydrated

One of the most common reasons for being unable to sleep through the night is dehydration. If you do not drink enough fluids throughout the day, your body will end up waking you up at night so that you can get a drink of water.

Additionally, not drinking enough water throughout the day may result in better sleep. This is because your body really needs water in order to function properly. One of the most important areas of the body that needs water is the brain.

By not keeping yourself hydrated, you are going to end up making your brain malfunction in a way. It will be unable to secrete the chemicals it is supposed to in order to help you fall asleep.

If you drink enough water throughout the day, your brain is going to be functioning at its optimal level. Hence, when you lay down to sleep you will have enough serotonin in your blood stream to help you shut down without having to toss and turn too much, and the chances of your sleep getting disturbed because your body needs water will become negligible.

Exercise at the Right Times

Exercise is widely accepted as one of the best ways to improve your sleep cycle. It regulates hormone levels in your body, boosts your bodies circulation thereby easing the strain and helping you to relax and it also helps to remove one of the biggest reasons for sleeplessness: stress.

However, exercising at the wrong time can get you into trouble too. If you exercise too late in the day, you may find yourself unable to sleep at the right time.

This is because when you exercise you fill your body with adrenaline. Adrenaline allows you to exert yourself more; it stimulates the heart and makes it pump faster so that your muscles can get oxygen at a faster rate. It also makes you extremely active, which is obviously not going to be very conducive to quality sleep.

The best time to exercise is early in the morning. If you can't exercise first thing in the morning, try to exercise any time before four pm. This is when a healthy body starts winding its various functions down, taking the brain on the long, slow crawl to sleep. If you exercise at this time, your body's shut down process will be interrupted.

Eat Light Dinners

You might have heard of the concept of taking a nap after a heavy meal. This is ostensibly true that one does feel quite sleepy after eating a hearty meal, but the problem with this is that the sleep you get after eating a big dinner is not conducive to a restful waking state.

If you eat a heavy dinner, your body is going to end up having to digest it. Digestion is a very active process. It involves a great deal of energy, and even if you don't know it's happening, your body is going to be busy metabolizing the food you have consumed.

This can make it difficult for you to fall asleep. After all, if your body is as active as it is while it is digesting heavy food, it certainly won't be able to reduce its internal functions to the point where it can ostensibly be referred to as "shut down".

Additionally, eating heavy meals only a few hours before bed is recipe for indigestion. Your body will be caught between the calm of sleep and the storm of digestion that will probably result in an aching stomach, something that can certainly cause you to wake up in the middle of the night.

Use as Much Natural Light as Possible

The problem with artificial lights is that they confuse our brains. We can recognize that these lights are fake but we sit in them for so long that we forget what natural light feels like.

Your brain can differentiate between real sunlight and the light that comes from artificial sources like bulbs to some extent. If you use as much natural light as possible while it is available, you are going to make it a lot easier for your brain to differentiate between it and artificial light.

This is going to make it a lot easier for you to sleep at night, as your brain will understand that the presence of fake light means that the sun has gone down.

In order to get as much natural light as possible, it is important that you keep your curtains open throughout the day, and go for walks while the sun is out. The light of the sun also helps to regulate your body's hormones, thus making it a lot easier for your body to secrete the chemicals that are necessary to facilitate quality sleep.

Get a Massage

If you have trouble falling asleep, try to get your significant other to give you a massage as part of your daily pre-sleep routine. Massages help relax your muscles, relieving them of the tension that has set in from hours of sitting in front of a computer screen at work.

Tense muscles as well as stress are two of the most important factors that can end up causing insomnia. This is because your body is unable to focus on shutting itself down if you are stressing out over something. Stress forces you to constantly think about the cause of your stress that makes it impossible for your brain to lower its activity to a level that would be conducive to sleep.

Tense muscles, on the other hand, cause old fashioned discomfort. They cause aches and pains that distract you from sleep. Hence, getting a massage that relieves your muscles of their tension is going to remove these distractions from your body.

Additionally, getting a massage stimulates the release of a chemical called serotonin in your brain that relaxes you. Filling your brain with this chemical will allow it to fall asleep more easily. The presence of this relaxing chemical also makes it easier for you to achieve REM sleep, which is the most relaxing kind of sleep.

Try this 5 minute self-massage in order to calm and relieve stress

-Begin by kneading the muscles located at the back of the neck and shoulders.

-Make a loose fist and then drum up and down the sides and the back of the neck

-Now use the thumbs to start working out tiny circles around the base of the head or skull.

-Use your fingertips to slowly massage the rest of the scalp. Tap the fingers against the scalp and move them from front to back, and later over the sides.

-Start to massage the face. Make a series of little circles using the fingertips or the thumbs. Pay attention to the jaw muscles, forehead, and the temples.

-Massage the bridge of your nose using the middle fingers, and progress to work outward on the eyebrows of the temples.

-Now close the eyes and cup the hand loosely over the face. Inhale and exhale easily for a moment.

- To make the massage more productive, incorporate massage oils such as almond essential oil.

With massage, you can also incorporate aromatherapy and decompressing techniques to gain the benefits of both worlds. You can incorporate massage with essential oils to relieve stress and other disturbing emotions that hinder effective sleep. Here you incorporate the sense of touch and the physical manipulation of muscles and joints. The sensation you get from massage together with the aroma from essential oils work together to release stress, anxiety, and worries. There are various ways of doing this:

-Apply almond, lavender or eucalyptus oil onto your hands and then breathe deeply into the oils.

-Also apply the oils onto your handkerchief, clothes or pillow or other stuff you can easily or regularly sniff

-Only get natural or unprocessed oils free from additives. Read the labels well to ensure that you obtain proper oils.

A warm decompress can also be used as a massage technique in order to relax your muscles and calm the mind. Just place a warm heat wrap around the neck and shoulders for around 10 minutes. Close the eyes and then relax the face, neck, back muscles, and the chest. Then remove the heat wrap and now use a foam roller or tennis ball to massage the tension away.

-Put the ball between the wall and your back.

-Lean into the ball, and then hold gentle pressure for about 10-20 seconds

-Now move the ball to a different spot and apply pressure in a similar manner

Write Down What's Worrying You

If you are stressed out about something and it's not letting you sleep, you need to get it out of your head. Constantly thinking about a specific topic is going to keep your brain extremely active, thus making it virtually impossible for you to fall asleep for long periods of time.

The best way to deal with this problem is to write down the thing that is causing you stress. Writing it down essentially brings it out of your head and onto a piece of paper. One it is written down, it is going to become something tangible, something that can be objectively analyzed.

When you have a thought in your head, it is essentially shapeless. Hence, it is difficult to deal with since your mind does not really know what the best course of action would be.

Writing your worry down gives it form. It turns it from something that you don't fully understand to something that you can read aloud to yourself. This can help you rationalize the thing that you are worrying about, for better or for worse, which will help you focus on sleeping instead of worrying.

On the other hand, there are other tips to help fight worries that affect your sleep:

1. Challenge anxious thoughts

The key here is to ensure you think positively in a manner to relax your mind and encourage sleep. Try to identify any challenging thought, and then brainstorm what scares you about the thought or event. For now, treat these details as plain hypothesis and then start to examine them to develop a more balanced perspective. After a careful examination of the situation, you will find more benefits of avoiding worries rather than accommodating them.

2. Evaluate available solutions

Evaluating the triggers of your worries should help you formulate ways of addressing them, and then put your strategic plan into action. Thus, you should distinguish between solvable and unsolvable worries, by evaluating whether the worry is real or just an imaginary "what-if", how likely the dreaded thing may occur and whether you can help in controlling the occurrence or outcome of the event.

Start by making a list of all available solutions through brainstorming. If the worries tend to be unsolvable, learn how to embrace your feelings. By doing this, you can easily experience anxiety episodes without being overwhelmed and later learn how to use them to your advantage.

3. Practice mindfulness

As worrying is usually pegged on the future, practicing mindfulness can assist you free your worries, and bring your attention back to the present. In this strategy, you don't have to postpone your worries, but instead face them boldly and let them go. You then find out how your thinking pattern results into worries, while still remaining in touch with your emotions. Practice these steps:

-Accept and study your anxious thoughts or feelings, without attempt to control, fight, or ignore them. Just view them as an outsider, without making any judgment or reaction.

-Allow your worries to go, by not engaging in them. You will find out that allowing the anxious thoughts to disappear on their own without any control over them, they just pass on their own

-Maintain your focus on the present by paying attention to your current feeling. Focus on your emotions, your rhythm of breathing, as well as those thoughts that interfere with your mind. When stuck on a particular thought, try to focus on it based on the present moment.

Take Herbal Teas To Help You Relax

Having a busy day and deadlines to beat can get you stressed and hinder an effective nap or good night sleep. Herbs like Chamomile and Valerian tea can help slow down the nervous system and offer relaxation you need. However, you need to consult a health expert before trying out herbs since some might interfere with other medications. If pregnant, nursing a baby or suffering from liver disease avoid herbs and embrace a glass of warm milk instead.

Try Getting Up Earlier

Everyone gets tempted. After last night difficult task, you'll feel more tempted to stay a little late in bed; which is a bad idea for everyone. If you sleep until late in the morning, this might interfere with your sleep schedule and occasional naps you take in the office. A good approach is to wake up at the same time everyday including weekends. Getting to or from bed at specific time can help form a rhythm and thus both your hormones and the mind will be prepared for sleep.

A better approach is to apply early-to-bed early-to-rise strategy in increments in a bid to train your body to anticipate sleep. Sleeping and waking up at the same time works for some people but can be harder to sustain if you're a night owl. You'll find out that to wake up at 6PM and later attempt to sleep by 12 AM is impossible, but if done through increments make a huge difference. So try to sleep 20 minutes earlier and wake up 20 minutes earlier.

Compared to just 'waking up earlier', doing it through increments is easy to sustain as you gradually train the body through a minor change. Actually, you won't even feel the 10-20 minutes difference. The following morning, adjust by another 10-20 minutes so that you'll wake up around 30 minutes earlier. Doing this a couple of weeks progressively can help you be a morning person within a month.

If you find waking up a challenge, try sleeping with the window open a crack if you bear it. Alternatively, have someone open the curtain or window to allow fresh air and natural daylight into the house. You can also invest in an Automatic Curtain Opener and set it to pen the drapes say 30 minutes earlier before the alarm clock. This experience stimulates your internal clock that it's time to get moving. In case the bedroom window's view is blocked, or doesn't have a window either, you can invest in a smart light that works through programming.

Animals or pets can be great alarm clocks, particularly for those that begin finding early in the morning. Remember that the recommended 8 hours of sleep is just an average than may vary from a person to another.

Be Mindful

Take a few minutes in your daily schedule to practice mindfulness, to help relax your body and mind. Once ready, close the eyes and then concentrate on your breathing. In case you have 10-20 minutes before taking a nap, go to a quiet environment, close your eyes and take a couple of deep breaths. Though you might not fall asleep immediately, mindfulness helps train your body to relax and get out of flight situation.

This breathing exercise is a good way of creating a relaxed mind and fall asleep quickly.

-Lie on a mat with the face up and arms positioned by your sides.

-Then bend the legs to about 90 degrees and lift the head and shoulders from the mat.

-Undertake 5 simultaneous inhales and follow these with 5 exhales.

-As you perform these, lift the arms from the mat and pulse them in unison with your breath palms facing up on inhale and down during exhale.

-Do these exercises about 10 times to undertake about 100 breaths.

When it comes to mindfulness, you don't have to follow many rules. However, there are the basics that help you effectively practice mindfulness and realize the results you really desire. Try to follow these simple guidelines:

1. Look for a quiet environment

Look for a secluded place either in the house, outdoors or in your office where you can easily relax without interruption or any distraction.

2. Be comfortable

Adopt a comfortable posture, but don't lie down as this might make you fall asleep. Ensure you sit with the spine straight, or be in lotus or cross-legged position.

3. Get a point of focus

Either with eyes open or closed, you can get mindful as far as you get a point of focus. This can be an object in your room, a candle, a mantra, or an imaginary scene.

4. Have the right attitude

You shouldn't care about stress or anxious thoughts that distract your mind. If any bad thought distracts you as you relax, don't fight the thoughts but get back to the point of focus.

A more recommended way to practice mindfulness is to visualize. Just sit up but you can also do it in any posture that can make you fall asleep during the process.

-Close the eyes and allow the worries to go away

-Visualize yourself in a glorious or calm place. Try to see a clear picture of where you are, based on what you can feel, see, hear, smell or taste.

-Choose an imagery that impresses you, only those images that work for you and not those you wish they impressed you.

-Try to incorporate as many sensory details as you can, so include at least 3 of your senses.

Spend some good time on each of your senses. Appreciate the feeling and the deep relaxation you achieve as you explore the restful place. Once ready, slowly open the eyes and get back to the present.

Relax Your Muscles

Ever heard of progressive muscle relaxation? This is a two-step process practice that allows you to tense and relax various muscles groups in your body. Being aware of how each tension feels like in your body can help you spot and control the initial signs of muscular tension that brings stress. You can easily learn to relax your body and mind, by combining deep breathing and muscle relaxation. In case you previously experienced back pain problems or muscle spasms, consult your doctor before trying this technique.

-Make yourself comfortable by loosening your outfit and removing the shoes

-Take some time to relax, by taking slow and deep breaths until you are ready to proceed

- Start by shifting your attention to the right foot, and take enough time to experience the way it feels

-Now tense the muscles in your right foot. Just squeeze the muscles as firm as possible, and then hold for a count of 10.

-Relax the right foot, and then focus on how tension flows away. Also experience how this foot feels as it turns limp and loose.

-Hold for a moment in this state, as you breathe deeply and very slowly

-After you are ready, you should then shift to your left foot. Repeat the same procedure to tense and release your muscles.

-Start to move gradually up through your body, as you contract and relax the muscle groups as you go. This practice may take some time before you get used to it, though regular training can really help.

Stop trying

Sleep is biological process that cannot be manipulated, so stop forcing sleep especially if you suffer from insomnia. On the other hand, trying to achieve sleep through medication has shown to worsen insomnia symptoms in the long-term. If you find sleeping or taking a nap harder, try to rest instead. Also don't attempt to compensate for any sleep lost as doing so might work against your natural sleep pattern and cause frustration.

Chapter 10: Common Sleep Misconceptions

Sleep is a heavily researched part of human biology, yet there are a number of mysteries and uncertainties still attached to it. With so much still unknown about sleep, misconceptions are bound to arise. Most of these misconceptions are harmless, but some might just be damaging to your health if you apply them to your daily sleep routine. In this chapter, the various myths associated with sleep will be discussed.

1. Sleeping is Just Being Unconscious

If you look at someone that is sleeping, you just see someone who has their eyes closed or someone who is basically doing nothing at all. When you sleep, you might not feel anything and you might not even dream. You'd just close your eyes and wake up a little while later feeling reasonably fresher than you did before.

Despite outer appearances, however, sleeping is not at all a passive activity, and it is a lot more than just being unconscious. While you are asleep, your brain is just as active as it is while you are awake. Your body is busy at work repairing itself and adjusting hormone levels until they have been optimized. This perception of sleep as a passive activity is what has lead to it being considered so unimportant, even though it is completely false.

2. You Need Less Sleep as You Grow Older

A lot of older people tend to wake up really early. Others stay up all night, claiming that they can't sleep. It is a common misconception that this is because old people in general don't feel as sleepy as younger people.

There are a number of diseases that can occur when a person gets old. Arthritis, diabetes, heart problems, all of these are things that any old person could potentially suffer from. However, just because that some, even most old people suffer from these diseases does not mean that it is inevitable that old people will get them. Not every old person will get arthritis, although a lot of them will.

The same goes for irregular sleep patterns. Some elderly individuals suffer from circadian rhythms disrupted by malfunctioning bodily functions, such as an enlarged prostate that is making it difficult to urinate, forcing you to get up in the middle of the night and ruining your sleep. You need just as much sleep as you always have when you grow older; it's just that it is possible that your body will become less effective at making you sleep than it used to be.

3. **You Can Deprive Yourself of Sleep and Catch Up on It Later**

This is a common process that people implement. They sleep four to six hours on weekdays and then sleep ten to twelve hours on weekends, thinking that this is going to allow them to "pay off" their sleep debt.

However, sleep doesn't work like that. You need a certain number of hours every single day otherwise your sleep debt will rise uncontrollably.

If you attempt to make up for lost sleep on the weekends, you might feel fresh at first but soon your sleep debt will be back. You will start the next week accumulating even more sleep debt while you already have a great deal of sleep debt to deal with already.

As this continued over a long period of time, eventually you are going to become sleep deprived, and the lack of sleep is going to start taking a toll on your body.

Stay on the safe side of things and just get a decent number of hours in every night. If you sleep more than six hours, you won't accumulate as much sleep debt and would be able to sleep it off over the weekend.

4. Snoring is a Normal Part of Sleep

People either believe in this misconception or they believe that snoring is a sign of very good sleep. After all, if someone is snoring it ostensibly means that they are in extremely deep sleep.

However, snoring is not normal and it is a long way off from being beneficial and a sign of good sleep. If you are snoring, it essentially means that one of your passageways is blocked, and the other one is only partially open which is what causes the loud snoring sound. This can cause minor symptoms such as a dry throat and a low chance of achieving REM sleep.

If this only happens once in a while it is not exactly healthy but not life threatening at all. However, if you are snoring extremely loudly and do it every night, it could be a sign of a serious illness known as sleep apnea. Sleep apnea can potentially result in death in a worst case scenario, so if you are snoring a lot go and see a doctor just in case.

5. Sleeping Pills are Fine to Use

A lot of people have trouble sleeping, and since we are used to getting instant results for our problems a lot of these people use sleeping pills to fall asleep. Using sleeping pills on a regular basis is widely considered to be an acceptable way to regulate your sleeping patterns.

However, sleeping pills can be quite harmful. First and foremost, sleeping pills could prevent your brain from falling asleep on its own. You would become too reliant on sleeping pills to fall asleep, which means that if you ever do not have a sleeping pill it might end up taking you hours to fall asleep.

Additionally, although sleeping pills do generally help you quickly fall asleep, the quality of sleep you get after taking a pill is highly inferior. You simply lose consciousness and regain it after a few hours, which mean that you are not exactly sleeping. Your body simply shuts down and does not perform any of the useful functions it does while you actually sleep.

Additionally, sleeping pills can cause complications such as heart palpitations, and can even increase the risk of cancer in some situations. When used very sparingly, sleeping pills can prove to be a useful cure for insomnia, but using them too often can make the side effects pile up and cause severe problems.

6. **You Don't Need More than Six Hours a Day**

With the amount of stress that people are under these days due to immense workloads, sleep has started to take a back seat in people's priorities increasingly often. People just don't feel that sleeping is a constructive use of their time, and they have so much work that they are unable to sleep for very long anyway.

As a result, a lot of people settle for four hours of sleep a day, thinking that this is enough to keep them going. For such people, six hours is the absolute maximum, thinking that six hours a day is more than enough to rest one's body and mind.

This is a dangerous misconception. Sleeping fewer than seven hours a day slowly increases sleep debt. If your daily sleep time is as low as four hours, you will find yourself horribly sleep deprived within a week, with a negative impact on your health hitting you hard. Make the time to sleep at least seven hours a night; it's worth it in the long run.

7. **Teenagers Sleep a Lot Because They are Lazy**

Teenagers have a tendency to sleep the day away, with many teenagers sleeping upwards of eight hours a day. Such teenagers often feel sleepy if they do not get at least eight to nine hours of sleep.

In today's culture where sleep deprivation is commonplace, such teenagers are viewed as lazy. This is also partly because of the general misconception that millenials are entitled and spoiled, despite the fact that they are growing up in the worst economy since the great depression.

The truth of the matter is, teenagers are going through a lot of changes in their bodies. One of the biggest changes has to do with their circadian rhythms. They start feeling sleepier later and later on during the day. This is not because they are lazy or want to stay up all night; it is because their body is naturally shifting its circadian rhythm around because of the hormonal havoc being wreaked by puberty.

Because of the way their body is changing, teenagers actually need more sleep than fully grown adults. Most teenagers need about nine to ten hours of sleep, as opposed to the seven to eight hours that the average adult needs. Hence, depriving a teenager of sleep can be even more dangerous than doing do to an adult, as teenagers need their rest a lot more than adults do.

If you have a teenage child, particularly a son, let them sleep in. As long as they are not actively trying to stay up late there is no reason to be worried about this. Their body will get used to the new hormones it is starting to secrete and by the time they hit nineteen or twenty they will start conforming to more adult sleeping patterns automatically.

8. **Waking up a Sleepwalker is Hazardous to Their Health**

This is a misconception that has somewhat uncertain roots. The origin may lie in folk tales that posited that people who sleepwalked were possessed by demons, due to the fact that sleepwalkers regularly talked and mumble incoherently while walking. As a result, people were discouraged from touching sleepwalkers.

This belief evolved over the years as people began to apply logic more and more often. It is still a common belief that sleepwalkers should not be disturbed, except that now people claim that this is because they can die from the shock of being woken up.

This is actually completely untrue. Sleepwalking does not have any medical implications that could result in death if they are awoken. Although it is not certain what exactly causes sleepwalking, it has been proven that sleepwalkers are not in danger of death if you disturb them.

Although it is possible that if you wake them up they will experience disorientation and confusion that might lead to stress, the vast majority of the time this stress is not nearly strong enough to cause a heart attack. The only situation where it is not a good idea to wake up a sleepwalker is if they have unconsciously walked into an extremely dangerous place, such as the roof of an apartment building.

9. Turkey Makes you Sleepy

The post Thanksgiving dinner naps that people tend to take popularized this myth. Since the main dish during thanksgiving is almost always turkey, people eventually started to assume that the reason post dinner festivities are dulled by drowsiness is that turkey contains some kind of chemical that can put you to sleep.

This belief was apparently legitimized when it was discovered that turkey contains a chemical that stimulates the production of serotonin, a hormone that calms you down and can make you drowsy. However, practically every white meat contains this chemical. Eating chicken, duck or fowl will most often cause the same secretion of serotonin in your brain. However, the amount of serotonin that is produced is not nearly enough to cause a lot of drowsiness.

The actual reason that people tend to get really sleeps after thanksgiving dinner actually has nothing to do with the type of meat that is eaten. Eating a great deal of protein can potentially cause drowsiness, as can the consumption of large amounts of carbohydrates.

Since you do eat large amounts of meat for Thanksgiving dinner, along with carb rich foods such as yams and potatoes, this is more likely what causes drowsiness. Additionally, Thanksgiving dinners tend to involve a great deal of alcohol. This exacerbates the drowsiness that is experienced after consuming so much protein.

Furthermore, our circadian rhythms tend to make us feel drowsy in the afternoon. Usually this drowsiness is not all that severe, as we do not have any chemicals present that can exacerbate it. However, on Thanksgiving your natural afternoon drowsiness is greatly compounded by large amounts of alcohol as well as protein and carbohydrates.

10. **Everyone Needs the Same Amount of Sleep**

Sleep experts tend to stand by the notion that everyone needs eight hours of sleep a day. While it is true that seven to eight hours has been recognized as the optimum duration of sleep for most people, there are a lot of people whose circadian rhythms greatly differ from the norm.

Sleep is a lot like eating. There are certain foods you can eat and certain foods you can't. Some people can eat enormous amounts of food, whereas other people can't really eat more than very small portions. There is a general consensus about how much a person should eat but there are people out there that still feel hungry after normal sized portions.

In the same way, a small percentage of people do not require more than six hours of sleep a day. For such people, sleeping eight hours will essentially be oversleeping which has its own adverse health effects attached to it.

Additionally, certain people tend to need an hour or so more than the traditional eight hours. Forcing themselves to sleep only eight hours will result in sleep debt accumulation.

11. **Sleeping Early is Healthy**

Benjamin Franklin, who claimed that waking up before the sun rose would be conducive to better health, popularized this misconception. A lot of people still believe that waking up early is an important part of maintaining one's health.

However, this philosophy holds no particular basis in truth. It is clear that Benjamin Franklin found that starting work as early as possible would result in the highest level of productivity. He probably could not concentrate at night and often found himself getting sleepy early.

This does not mean that everyone should follow the exact same routine. What worked for Benjamin Franklin might not work for you. If you are naturally inclined to sleep early then do so by all means. However, there is a chance that you might find yourself at your most productive late at night. You might feel inclined to sleeping during the day. There is absolutely nothing wrong with this.

The only thing that you need to take care of is regularity. Whatever your sleep schedule is, whether you are an early bird or a night owl, just keep your sleep timings consistent. You need to go to sleep ever sixteen to seventeen hours for eight to seven hours.

12. Energy Drinks are a Great Way to Stay Awake

People these days are obsessed with sleeping as less as possible. This is why so many people consume energy drinks in order to stay awake longer. These energy drinks contain large amounts of caffeine, and can ostensibly help keep you awake for long periods of time.

However, these drinks contain enormous amounts of sugar. This sugar will boost your caffeine high, making you feel alert for a short while. However, once the sugar has been metabolized you are going to end up crashing. Your body will get twice as tired as it was before because it was unable to get rest when it really needed it.

The better option in these situations would be coffee. At least in coffee you are only going to be consuming at most a tablespoon of sugar with your required dose of caffeine.

If you need to stay up late, try drinking a cup of coffee or tea instead of chugging down an energy drink. Apples are also excellent ways to stay awake, and are a lot healthier than both tea and coffee, and are obviously a lot healthier than energy drinks.

13. **Cheese Before Bed Results in Bad Dreams**

This is another myth that has been popularized by television and movies. There are many instances of television episodes where a character eats cheese and falls asleep, only to suffer from vivid and terrifying nightmares. The first ever instance where cheese was associated with bad dreams was in the story "A Christmas Carol", in which the main character is told that the dreadful nightmares he is suffering from is being caused by his love for cheese.

In fact, this has actually become true for a lot of people. Certain people do end up suffering from vivid nightmares while they sleep. However, this is not because of the cheese per se. The people who react badly to cheese and end up suffering from nightmares are usually on anti depressants. Anti depressants fill your body with chemicals that do not react well with cheese.

This results in disruptions in your mental chemistry that eventually causes bad dreams when you go to sleep. For the vast majority of people, eating cheese before you sleep is not going to cause any bad dreams whatsoever. However, if you are on anti depressants, avoid the cheese if you want a good night's sleep.

14. **Sleepiness during Driving is Easily Cured**

It is a common misconception that if you are feeling sleepy while driving, all you need to do is roll down the window. The wind will keep you fresh and alert.

Another commonly recommended cure for sleepiness while driving is turning some music on. The logic here is that music will keep your brain engaged, thus making it difficult for you to fall asleep. If the music that you are listening to is high in volume, you will be unable to sleep because of the noise.

However, these tips are based on the assumption that sleepiness while driving is no different from any other kind of sleepiness. This is completely untrue. If you are getting sleepy while performing a task that is as active as driving, it means that you are extremely sleep deprived.

You are sleep deprived to the point where your brain has started shutting down automatically because it simply cannot take any more work without resting first.

The only way to prevent accidents caused by sleepiness while driving is to never drive while you are in this state. Stay well rested, and if you are sleepy just take a taxi home. Driving simply isn't worth the risk.

15. You Can Only Dream During the Rapid Eye Movement Phase of Sleep

You have probably studied in school about the REM portion of sleep. During this phase of sleep, your eyes will be moving underneath your eyelids. It is during this phase of sleep that dreams occur.

This is actually a misconception based loosely on fact. During REM sleep, your brain is at its most active out of any other period of sleep. This is because you are dreaming at your most vivid. Most often, the dreams that you remember when you wake up are the dreams that you were having during REM sleep.

However, this does not mean that you are not dreaming at all outside of REM sleep. Dreams occur at random period throughout your sleep session. The only difference between these dreams and the dreams you see during REM sleep is that these dreams are usually mundane and are very rarely remembered.

Dreams experienced during REM sleep can be fantastical and psychedelic, and thus leave a deeper impression that might cause you to remember the dream after you wake up.

16. You Yawn When you are Tired

Yawning is associated with sleep. Whenever somebody yawns,

it is usually considered to be a sign that your body requires sleep. This is because of a misconception regarding why we yawn that a lot of people believe.

This misconception is that we yawn because our body is trying to get as much oxygen as possible in order to stay awake, as it is assuming that you need to stay up since you are not already asleep. This clearly does not make sense. If yawning were a way for the body to oxygenate itself more efficiently, we would start yawning after exerting ourselves not panting and gasping.

Yawning actually has nothing to do with sleep itself; its function is hypothesized to be entirely different. Although it is not exactly certain why we yawn, research has shown that yawning cools down the blood that is in our face. This cooling effect relaxes us. This is why you might find yourself yawning at some point during the day. You might end up feeling relaxed and sleepy because of the yawn.

Hence, yawning, not the other way around causes drowsiness. We tend to yawn a lot before we sleep because our body cools down while it is preparing for a sleep session. In order to facilitate a rapid reduction in body temperature around the face, it makes you yawn. This also acts as a signal that your body is ready for sleep if the need arises.

Hence, if you are yawning a lot during the day don't worry. This does not mean that you are sleep deprived or that you need sleep at that very moment. The drowsiness is just because yawning makes you feel comfortable. Just have a coffee or tea and you will be active again in no time.

17. **Warm Milk Acts as a Sedative**

We've all heard of this one. If you are having trouble falling asleep, just have a glass of warm milk before bed and you will be out like a light.

The scientific evidence that milk may help us sleep is that it contains an amino acid that stimulates the production of serotonin. However, much as is the case with turkey, the amount of serotonin that milk produces is not nearly enough to help you fall asleep if you are not already sleepy.

However, a lot of people report that having a glass of warm milk definitely helps them to sleep easier at night. Scientific studies have shown a definite correlation between sleeping easily and drinking warm milk. However, this has nothing whatsoever to do with the effect that milk has biologically.

More likely, drinking milk reminds you of your childhood and allows you to enter a state of mind similar to when you were a baby still breastfeeding. The psychological impact that drinking milk has probably makes you feel relaxed. Hence, warm milk is essentially a placebo rather than a substance that has a genuine sedating effect on your body.

If you are looking for something you can eat that will make you feel sleepy, try eating foods rich in carbohydrates. Carbohydrates are broken down into glucose. The excess glucose in your bloodstream prompts your pancreas to release insulin that turns this glucose into fat.

This process of converting glucose to fat produces an enormous amount of serotonin that will help you fall asleep extremely easily. Hence, if you are having troubles sleeping just have some carbohydrate rich foods about half an hour before bedtime and you will be out like a light.

18. Counting Sheep Helps You Sleep

This is yet another misconception that has been brought about by its prevalence in popular culture. Counting sheep refers to an activity where you count the number of sheep that are jumping over a fence. This activity is highly mundane and boring, which is ostensibly supposed to allow you to fall asleep quickly if you are having trouble doing so.

By counting sheep, you are supposedly able to distract yourself from stressors and other thoughts that might be forcing you to stay awake.

However, the problem with counting sheep is that it is perhaps too mundane. If you count sheep, you won't really be occupying that much of your brain. Since counting sheep is so easy, your brain will be able to continue focusing on the problems that are causing you stress.

In fact, counting shape may even make it even more difficult for you to fall asleep. As repetitive as the activity is, it does utilize your brain albeit in a miniscule amount. The fact that your brain is active is going to make it difficult for it to shut down. It will slow down the process of falling asleep. On average, people that count sheep take almost half an hour longer to sleep than people who don't.

19. Insomniacs Should Never Drink Coffee

Insomnia is a very serious disease that affects a large number of people. Insomniacs are basically people who are unable to sleep no matter how tired they are. There are a number of causes for insomnia, the most common being stress, but a lot of people mistakenly associate the consumption of coffee with insomnia.

The logic is sound enough. The caffeine in coffee makes you active. However, it is all about the timing of your coffee consumption. Consuming coffee less than four hours before you try to sleep can result in difficulty falling asleep.

However, consuming coffee at any other time during the day will not result in insomnia. Coffee gets processed and metabolized fairly quickly. The caffeine gives you a quick buzz that can last for about two hours, after which you will either go back to normal or will experience a minor crash. By this time, your body has removed all the caffeine from within itself via your urine.

Hence, if you are suffering from insomnia, there is absolutely no reason that you should avoid coffee, as long as you are drinking it more than four hours before you have to go to bed.

20. Sleeplessness Can be Cured by Staying in Bed

This is a common technique that people use. If they are unable to fall asleep, they just stay in bed and keep their eyes shut, hoping that sleep will eventually come.

This is never effective. If you stay wake in bed, your mind will eventually stop associating your bed with being a place of sleep. This is only going to exacerbate your insomnia.

If you are unable to sleep, the best thing that you can do is get out and do something else. Try reading a book while sitting on the sofa, or listening to some relaxing music. Try doing things that might make you drowsy instead of just laying in bed.

21. Dreams Serve No Purpose

Most of us do not understand the importance of dreams. We tend to think of dreams as random, disjointed pictures that are just the product of our brain sorting through the memories of the previous day.

This is entirely untrue. Dreams serve an extremely important function. Over the course of our lives, we end up wanting a lot of things that we can't get. We also suffer traumas and go through bad experiences that we try to forget.

Both of these things are made easier to deal with because of dreams. In a dream, you might see yourself achieving something that you weren't able to achieve in real life. This will help you to not to feel so disappointed when you are unable to get what you want in real life.

Dreams also play an important role in helping us deal with trauma and grief. We experience our traumas and bad experiences often in fantastical or embellished scenarios. This is our sleeping mind rationalizing and processing emotions that the waking mind cannot.

Chapter 11: Little Known Facts About Sleep

1. You Sleep Better During the Full Moon (And Worse during New Moons)

This is a rather odd and inexplicable fact about sleep. It has been noticed in a number of people who claim that whenever the full moon is out, they tend to sleep better. These people report more restful sleep as well as more vivid dreams. On the other hand, sleeping during the new moon is often fraught with bad dreams and sleep paralysis. It is as yet unknown if this is an anomaly or if the lunar cycle actually has a tangible effect on our sleep.

2. It Should Take You Ten to Fifteen Minutes to Fall Asleep

When you rest your head to sleep, you are probably going to take about ten to fifteen minutes until you finally descend into true, deep slumber. This is because it takes your brain this long to recognize that it is time to properly shut down. If it takes you less than ten minutes to fall asleep, or if you fall asleep as soon as your head hits the pillow, it means that you are suffering from sleep deprivation. Try to increase the number of hours you sleep if this is the case.

3. Peak Sleep Can be Attained at Two Different Times during the Day

If you need further proof that night owls are not leading unhealthy lives, you should know that you can experience deepest sleep at two in the morning and two in the afternoon. This is why you often feel drowsy in the afternoon. If you are the type of person that sleeps during the day, two hours after midday is going to be when you are sleeping your deepest and seeing your most vivid dreams. If you are an early bird, don't worry if you feel drowsy in the afternoon. It is a natural part of your circadian rhythm.

4. Weekend Schedules Make Mondays Harder

Being unable to wake up on Monday is not just caused by the thought of having to go to work. Most of us tend to alter our sleep patterns during the weekend. We go out with our friends and party until it's late, we stay up all night watching movies, and some of us just stay up with a book.

This common adjustment that many of us make to our sleep patterns over the weekend disrupts our circadian rhythms, and our minds struggle to wake up early on Monday as a result.

5. No Other Animal Willingly Delays Sleep

We have become so tied up in this consumer culture where we are constantly told to work harder to live better that we don't realize what we are sacrificing to gain the fleeting satisfaction of consumption. We ignore the health problems caused by sleeplessness because we have so many distractions that give us instant gratification. No other animal on Earth willingly avoids or delays sleep apart from humans because they instinctively know that doing so will cause major health problems.

6. There Are Many Causes for Insomnia

Although it is widely believed that insomnia is caused only by stress, there are several other factors that could go into it. You might have inadequate sleeping arrangements that are not conducive to restful sleep, you might be suffering from a physical or mental illness that is preventing you from falling asleep easily or your insomnia might be the result of a poor diet. Insomnia can also be caused by employment at places where you are required to work in shifts. These shifts wreak havoc with your circadian rhythm and make it difficult for you to maintain a regular sleep schedule.

7. An Inability to Get Out of Bed May be an Actual Condition

A condition known as dysania makes it difficult for you to get out of bed in the morning. You might feel a lack of motivation or that your sleep needs are never adequately fulfilled. Dysania is often a symptom of depression, and if you are experiencing it this could mean that your depression is getting serious. Dysania can also be caused by an improper diet, as your body will not be able to differentiate between sleep and wakefulness easily due to hormonal imbalances.

8. Insomnia Doesn't Mean Lack of Sleep

When most people think of insomnia, they tend to assume that it is a condition that makes it difficult to fall asleep. Insomnia is actually not defined by how much you sleep each night. Rather, it is defined by the quality of your sleep. If you are experiencing poor sleep quality, you might be feeling irritable or drowsy the next day no matter how much you sleep. If this is the case then it is possible that you are suffering from a mild form of insomnia. You may be sleeping six to eight hours and still be suffering from insomnia.

9. Sleep Deprivation is Similar to Intoxication

Once you have been awake for sixteen hours in a row, your cognitive performance will begin to steadily decline. In fact, after being awake for sixteen hours your cognitive performance will actually be comparable with that of someone who has consumed a beer or two. After you have been awake for eighteen hours in a row, you will have the cognitive performance of someone who has a blood alcohol level of around 0.08%, which is the legal limit. This is why driving while sleep deprived is so dangerous and can result in accidents similar to those that occur while driving intoxicated.

10. Sleeping in One Go is a Recent Development

For a large chunk of human history, a lot of people would not sleep in one long block. In Europe up until the seventeenth century, people would sleep for around three to four hours, wake up for around an hour and then go back to sleep.

They would use this hour of wakefulness to study or to pray.

Some people even used this time to meet friends or spend time with family. It is unknown why this was the way people slept, but most research indicates that it had something to do with the fact that prayer was recommended during the earliest hours of the morning, and people would get up for an hour at this time in order to accommodate their religious beliefs.

Although this type of sleep pattern is no longer prevalent among Christians, Muslims who pray at the break of dawn still commonly practice it. It is common for Muslims even today to sleep for a few hours, wake up for an hour to pray and then sleep for another few hours.

This goes to show how many different types of sleep cycles there are.

11. Sleep Deprivation Often Makes you Hungry

You might find that when you go long periods of time without sleep, you are going to start feeling hungrier. This is essentially caused by hormonal imbalances in your body. As you already know, there are several functions that your body performs while you are asleep. One of the most important is the regulation of your hormones.

If you are sleep deprived, it means that your body has not had the opportunity regulate hormone levels. As a result, you are going to end up with low levels of one particular hormone called leptin. This is the hormone that is responsible for regulating your appetite.

If your body is functioning normally, it will secrete leptin after you have eaten in order to suppress your appetite. This is done in order to prevent you from over eating. However, if you haven't been getting enough sleep, your body will essentially be too tired to regulate the secretion of leptin.

Hence, you are not going to feel the same suppression of appetite after you are full and are going to end up feeling hungry more often. It is not exactly one of the worst side effects of sleep deprivation but it can cause weight gain if you are not careful.

12. Traffic Accidents Decrease with Daylight Savings

Daylight savings is a rather antiquated custom that involves turning the clocks back one hour so that you have one extra hour of daylight every day. Daylight savings actually decreases the number of traffic accidents that occur. This is because people end up getting an additional hour of sleep. As a result, they are less likely to be sleep deprived which ends up greatly decreasing the chances of being involved in an accident.

13. Waking People Up Used to Be a Job

Being unable to wake up for work is not a modern development. People have always found it difficult to wake up when they face a day of work and toil ahead of them. This is a natural psychological response. While sleeping we are at our most comfortable. Our serotonin levels skyrocket and we experience a feeling of contentment.

Work, on the other hand, represents just that: work. When that comes at the expense of sleep, it makes it extremely difficult for you to get out of bed.

This is why not all that long ago, when the industrial revolution kicked in and the process of manufacturing had started to get streamlined, some people were paid to wake employees up for work.

Their job was to go around to where workers' lived about half an hour before work was supposed to begin and ensure that they were awake. It would be safe to assume that these people were probably the most hated employees in the company.

14. The Japanese Frequently Sleep at Work

Falling asleep at work in most countries is a sign of laziness. After all, you are supposed to be doing your job, not catching up on sleep. Hence, if you are caught sleeping on the job you are probably going to be thought of as irresponsible.

This is the exact opposite of how sleeping at work is looked at in Japan. The Japanese view sleeping at work as the sign of a hard worker. If a manager sees that his or her employee is asleep at their desk, they would assume that it was because said employee had worked himself to the point of exhaustion that would earn them major points. Clearly the Japanese are far too honest to sleep at work if they are not tired in order to gain brownie points.

15. You Need to Guarantee That You Will Remain Well Rested Before Renting a Car

Driving while deprived of sleep is such a huge problem that some car rental companies make people who want to rent their cars sign a contract stating that they are going to rent the car on the condition that they won't sleep less than six hours a night.

This was put into place because driving while deprived of sleep had started to cause a lot of accidents, resulting in major financial loss for a lot of car rental companies.

16. Taking Sleeping Pills to Cure Insomnia Can Be Harmful

A lot of people think that insomnia is a disease that can be treated with medicine just like any other illness. However, insomnia is not an illness; it is a symptom. If you are suffering from insomnia, chances are that your body needs you to stay awake.

An example of such a situation is during the grieving process. If you have lost a loved one or have gone through some major trauma, you are probably not going to be able to get a decent amount of sleep. Your brain will just be too consumed with grief to shut down.

Hence, a lot of people take sleeping pills to cure their insomnia. This is actually the worst thing you can do. Sleeping pills induce unconsciousness, not actual sleep. The unconscious state you descend into after taking sleeping pills is not restful at all. Your body cannot repair itself the way it does during real sleep.

As a result, you are going to wake up with a disrupted circadian rhythm and none of the benefits that can be derived from actual sleep. This will make it even more difficult for you to get over your insomnia, because you are going to start accumulating sleep debt.

17. **Regular Exercise is Good for Sleep, Sporadic Exercise is Not**

If you have a regular exercise routine, chances are that your sleep cycle is going to be regular and will provide you with quality sleep. However, exercising irregularly tends to have the opposite effect.

If you exercise sporadically, your body is going to end up getting confused about when to secrete adrenaline. This is going to end up making it difficult to fall asleep as your hormone levels are going to be disrupted and irregular.

18. **The Rise of Colored Television Affected Our Dreams**

A rather unusual fact about sleep has to do with the effect that colored television had on our dreams. The exact reason for this is unknown, but being able to see dreams in color before color television was introduced was considered exceptional. Only around one in six people were able to see dreams in real color. Everybody else only ever saw black and white dreams.

However, all of this changed when colored television started to become commonplace. People began to see colored dreams more and more often. However, everybody does not see even nowadays colored dreams. About one in four people still see dreams in either very dull color or in black and white.

Researchers are perplexed as to what could have caused this

massive increase in the number of people who were able to see colored dreams. One researcher posited that watching colored television allowed our brains to recognize colors in a subconscious or unconscious state.

However, researchers have not been able to understand why exactly we were not able to see dreams in color before color television became commonplace.

19. The Biggest Cause of Insomnia is Neither Stress nor Caffeine

Our biggest source of sleeplessness has nothing to do with stress inducing events in our lives, nor does it have anything to do with the amount of coffee that we consume. It has to do with an aspect of our lives that we are so addicted to, we don't even know how addicted we are. Addiction to this thing has become commonplace, and is seen in children as young as twelve.

The biggest cause of insomnia is actually the internet. Or rather, perpetual access to the internet is what causes insomnia. We have become so used to spending all of our time surfing through our virtual lives that we have stopped paying attention to important aspects of our real lives.

The internet's ability to consistently provide instant gratification keeps our brains consistently active. The constant craving for the internet and all of the virtual comfort it provides makes it difficult for us to fall asleep easily.

This does not mean that you should restrict your access to the internet. It just means that you should avoid using the internet about an hour before sleep. Try turning your phone off in order to make it as difficult as possible for you to give in to temptation.

20. You Will Spend a Third of Your Life Sleeping

Most people don't realize just how much time we spend sleeping. Although all of the time we spend sleeping is essential and vital to living a healthy life, the fact remains that we spend decades of our lives sleeping.

If you maintain a consistent sleep schedule and get the prescribed number of hours every night, you are going to end up sleeping around two decades over the course of your life at least, assuming that you die of natural causes when you are old. This could even go up to almost three decades if you sleep a lot.

21. **This Number Will Be Higher If You Don't Have Children**

Having a child will inevitably result in a great many sleepless nights. Children demand attention, and this means that you are frequently woken up in the middle of the night, and will often have to spend several hours each night trying to get your crying baby to go to sleep.

As a result, most parents end up missing out on the equivalent of half a year of sleep while their baby is still an infant. Hence, not having a baby would allow you to sleep more in the long run, though many people would consider this emotionally unfulfilling.

22. **These Numbers Are Nothing When You Compare Them to Cats**

You might be surprised that humans spend a third of their lives sleeping. However, we practically spend our entire lives awake if we compare how much we sleep to how much cats sleep.

Cats spend a whopping seventy percent of their lives sleeping. If you spent an equivalent amount of time sleeping, you would probably be asleep for over half a century!

23. **The Amount of Time Giraffe's Sleep is Ridiculous**

Human beings sleep for a third of their lives sleeping, whereas cats spend three quarters of their lives sleeping. Giraffes, on the other hand, only sleep a measly two percent of their lives.

They tend to sleep no more than thirty minutes every day, with most giraffes able to get by with just five or so minutes of sleep a day.

Studies are being conducted using giraffe genes and hormones in an attempt to create a substance that would allow people to remain healthy while eliminating the need to sleep.

24. The Longest Period of Time Anyone Has Ever Gone Without Sleep is Amazing

You might have wondered how long you could possible go without sleeping. One man actually tried to see for himself. He went almost two weeks without sleep, an astounding eleven days to be exact. He did not suffer from any major negative health effects, although he had difficulty concentrating for longer than a minute or two towards the end of it, and ended up sleeping sixteen hours in a row after he was done.

25. Deaf People Talk in Their Sleep

Many people talk in their sleep. It is just the way some of us process the emotions that we are feeling. However, deaf people also talk in their sleep, and in sign language to boot.

This goes to show that when we talk in our sleep, we are actually communicating in some way instead of just muttering random sounds and words. Deaf people are known to speak entire sentences in sign language and since sign language is impossible to mishear, it makes it easier to study what people talk about when they speak while asleep.

26. You Never Sneeze While Sleeping

Sneezing is a way for your body to clear out your sinuses and to expel dust and bacteria that might have gotten in through the nose. However, we never sneeze while sleeping. This is because sneezing is a highly active process. If something makes you sneeze, the force of the sneeze will end up awakening you. Otherwise, the body shuts down processes that lead to things like sneezes so that it can focus on the various tasks it performs while you are asleep.

27. Lack of Sleep is Far More Dangerous than Starvation

You would never deprive yourself of food, yet if your work or personal life demanded it, you would gladly deprive yourself of sleep. However, you might think twice after you realize just how much more dangerous a lack of sleep is than starvation.

You can survive without any food for around two months as long as you have water. That is a pretty long period of time. You would start suffering reversible negative health consequences after about a week of hunger and after a month of starvation the toll it will have put on your body by now will be near irreversible, but if you are able to eat after two months, you will be able to survive.

You cannot survive beyond a mere two weeks if you do not sleep. You will begin to suffer from reversible negative health consequences within about a day and a half without sleep, and after four days you will start inflicting permanent damage on your body. Two weeks is the upper limit. Most people die after being deprived of sleep for about ten days.

This is how important sleep is. Your body can simply start consuming your body fat and eventually your muscles if you are not eating anything for a long period of time. It will adapt to the situation in order to keep you alive for as long as possible. However, your body simply cannot adapt to not getting any sleep. Sleep is the bare minimum requirement for staying alive.

28. Sleeping Helps Lose Weight in Other Ways Too

You already know that sleeping helps you lose weight by facilitating the regulation of your hormones. However, this is not the only way in which sleep helps you to keep your weight down.

A recent study discovered that you burn more calories while sleeping than while watching TV. So swap that TV time for a nap and get healthier while losing more weight in the process!

29. You Didn't Always Dream

Dreams are an important part of the maintenance of your health, but you did not dream since your life first began. Babies start dreaming properly after the age of three. This is because before they are there they simply do not have the memory to retain any experiences.

Since they never remembered any of their experiences, they would not have any material with which to dream. Additionally, babies younger than three are essentially emotionless. They have not developed the capacity for emotion yet. Once the capacity for emotion develops, they start having feelings that they need to rationalize which leads to them having dreams.

30. Women Dream More than Men

It is unknown why exactly this is so, but women tend to dream more than men. Their dreams also tend to be more vivid and emotionally charged, with the primary emotions usually being ones like sadness. Men, on the other hand, tend to experience fear more often during their dreams, as well as embarrassment.

However, despite the male tendency to experience more fear in dreams than women, women tend to have more dreams that could be classified as proper nightmares.

31. There Has Been a Person Who Didn't Need Sleep

In the Second World War, a man who had been fighting for the Hungarian army was shot in the head. The bullet went right through his frontal lobe but he miraculously survived. However, he found that he absolutely could not fall asleep anymore after that incident. He never slept again in his life.

This man is the only person in history to have gone longer than two weeks without sleeping and survived. In fact, this man lived out his life with little to not negative health consequences. For all intents and purpose, he lived a long and healthy life despite the fact that he had never been able to sleep.

32. The Removal of Light Changes Sleep Patterns Dramatically

Studies have been conducted where individuals have been subjected to environments that are perpetually dark in order to see the affect this would have on their circadian rhythms.

With no light to guide their brains, their bodies began to adjust to a very specific sleep schedule. These people began staying awake for around thirty six hours and then sleeping for twelve. Hence, their bodies automatically adjusted themselves to conform to a forty eight hour cycle rather than the traditional twenty four hour cycle. It was unclear why this phenomenon occurred.

33. It is Possible to Control Your Dreams

Some people are able to exert some form of control over their dreams. This is known as lucid dreaming. Lucid dreaming can allow you to ostensibly live out whatever fantasy you choose while you are still asleep and dreaming.

It is unknown if lucid dreams can be controlled to the extent where you can do anything in your dreams. The most people have been able to achieve so far has been becoming aware that they are dreaming. However, it has been theorized that if lucid dreaming is taken to a level where complete control is made possible, people can use these dreams to get over traumatic experiences.

There are several ways in which you can start lucid dreaming. One of the most popular ways is to start writing a dream diary. This basically involves writing down whatever you can remember about your dream as soon as you wake up. This will initially help you to start remembering your dreams more often. You will eventually be able to recall more details about your dreams.

This will allow you to recognize the themes and motifs that

recur in your dreams. Hence, when you are actually in a dream and start seeing these motifs and themes, you are going to become aware of the fact that you are actually asleep. This is the first step to lucid dreaming.

Once you become adept at recognizing when you are in a dream, you will eventually be able to control yourself inside your dream. The goal is to be able to make your dream bend to your will, so that while you are dreaming there is nothing that you can't do. This will allow you to get over traumatic events by molding your dream to represent them and taking control.

Playing video games is also an excellent way to start having lucid dreams. While you are playing a video game, you are essentially controlling an avatar in a virtual world. This is actually not so different from controlling yourself while lucid dreaming.

If you are maintaining a dream diary and are working your way towards becoming self aware while dreaming, try playing video games at the same time as well. The dream diary will help you to become self aware, while the video games will help make it easier for you to control yourself when you become self aware.

Conclusion

With these life hacks and strategies in place, you will find that your nightly rest is becoming a natural part of your routine. Instead of lying awake, your mind restlessly reviewing the events of the day and its challenges, you will be drifting off to sleep with ease.

Because of your newly enhanced sleep life, lived out in your dedicated sanctuary, you will be waking up feeling more refreshed and rested; ready to take on the day.

Your new life habits, having become intimate friends and supports, are leading you to better health, productivity and the kind of positive attitude that people respond to. That means a better life for you, lived more fully.

Don't be surprised if people look at you and tell you that you look rested, refreshed and maybe even younger!

Because you've taken control of your life and taken back your time, you're now feeling better than you've felt in a very long time.

The power of a good night's sleep is now yours. Sleep well, my friends! Feel amazing!

BONUS

Sleep is just one aspect of your health, and I am certainly glad you started there. If you are interested is taking your health (and life ultimately!) to the next level, I recommend the guide below to learn other easy-to-follow techniques you can apply today!

<u>FREE BONUS:</u> <u>23 Health Tips & Hacks You Probably Aren't Doing But Should Be to Reduce Fatigue, Improve Sleep and Recovery, Boost Sex Drive, and Heal Your Gut</u>

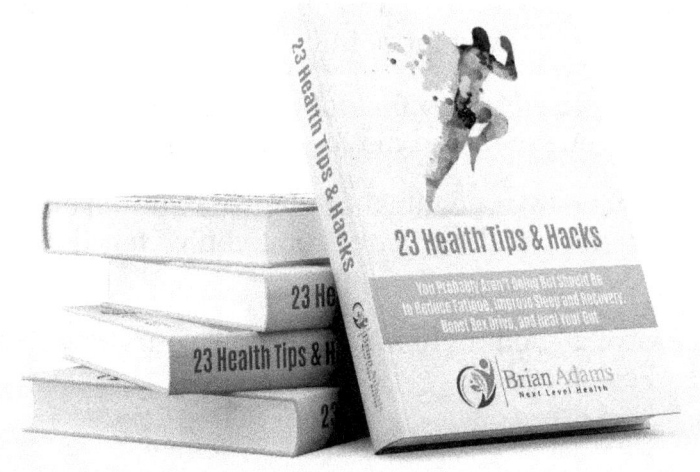

Link: https://publishfs.leadpages.co/getultrahealth/

P.S. Check out my other books too if you found this one helpful.

Recommended Reading

Achieve Your Next Level Health With a Click Away:

Low Carb: Ketogenic Diet to Overcome Belly Fat, Lose Pounds, and Live Healthy

Health and Fitness: Uncommon HIGH Impact Quick Wins You Should Start Today - Nutrition, Natural Health, and Healthy Living

Intermittent Fasting: Shortcut to Build Muscle, Lose Fat, and Easy Weight Loss

Detox: Cleanse for Fast Weight Loss, Anti Aging, Holistic Healing and Better Health

Vegan: Vegan Diet for Easy Weight Loss and Healthy Living Through Natural Foods

Other Recommended Books to Become More Effective and Fulfilled In Life:

Self Improvement: Self Discipline - An Uncommon Guide to Instant Self Control, Incredible Willpower, and Insane Productivity

Spirit Guides: Ultimate Guide to Exploring the Spirit World, Finding Your Angel Guide and Mastering Spirit Communication

Resources

The National Sleep Foundation is a wellspring of information on sleep, sleeping disorders and research: https://sleepfoundation.org/

The Center for Disease Control and Prevention has a section of their site entirely dedicated to sleeping and sleep disorders: http://www.cdc.gov/sleep/index.html

The Mayo Clinic Sleep Medicine Centers: These can be found in a number of US States. This link is a good place to start: http://www.mayoclinic.org/diseases-conditions/sleep-disorders/care-at-mayo-clinic/why-choose-mayo-clinic/con-20037263

Find out everything you'd like to know about yoga at this helpful resource: https://yoga.com/

Just what it says it is – a world of swimming information: http://www.swimmingworldmagazine.com/

A fun video of a water pole dancing class: https://www.youtube.com/watch?v=_Xl1j5Gt19Q

This is a handy introduction aquafit, detailing some of its routines: https://www.youtube.com/watch?v=cBbA4-EhNf8

The world is your playground, with geo-caching:

https://www.geocaching.com/play

An introduction to Dr. Weil's 4-7-8 breathing technique for better sleep: http://www.drweil.com/drw/u/VDR00112/The-4-7-8-Breath-Benefits-and-Demonstration.html

Snoring therapies can be found at this Mayo Clinic link. Again, a great starting point: http://www.mayoclinic.org/diseases-conditions/snoring/basics/definition/con-20031874